Manual of
HYDROTHERAPY AND MASSAGE

Manual of Hydrotherapy and Massage

Fred B. Moor, B.A., M.D.
Professor of Physical Medicine and Rehabilitation
School of Medicine
Medical Director, School of Physical Therapy
Loma Linda University
Los Angeles, California

Stella C. Peterson, B.S., R.N., A.R.P.T.
Instructor in Physical Therapy
School of Physical Therapy
Loma Linda University
Loma Linda, California

Ethel M. Manwell, B.S., R.N., A.R.P.T.
Chief Physical Therapist, Rheumatic Disease Clinic
White Memorial Medical Center
Los Angeles, California

Mary C. Noble, B.S., R.N., A.R.P.T.
Chief Physical Therapist
Paradise Valley Sanitarium and Hospital
National City, California

Gertrude Muench, R.N., R.P.T.
Chief Physical Therapist
Florida Sanitarium and Hospital
Orlando, Florida

PACIFIC PRESS PUBLISHING ASSOCIATION
Mountain View, California
Oshawa, Ontario

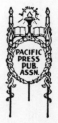

Dedicated to the memory of

===

Dr. George Knapp Abbott

Christian physician,

teacher, author,

proponent of scientific

physical therapy

PREFACE

This manual is presented as a teaching aid in the instruction of students in schools of nursing and physical therapy. The physician who writes the prescription for hydrotherapy or massage must entrust its actual application to the nurse or the physical therapist. He should have the assurance that those who execute his prescription are well qualified. Although the administration of hydrotherapeutic procedures is not technically difficult, good results are dependent upon meticulous attention to detail. Massage is an art which requires diligent practice to develop the finesse for which every conscientious student should strive. Therefore, the therapist (nurse or physical therapist) should endeavor to develop a faultless technique in both hydrotherapy and massage. This is acquired first by practice in the laboratory and later by closely supervised treatment of patients. Even as education in any field of learning does not end on commencement day, so the therapist should aim for perfection of technique after his formal training is completed.

But technical skill is not enough; the therapist should know the underlying physical and physiological principles. He should know the properties of the physical agents he is using—in this instance, water. He should be familiar with the local and general effects of heat and cold upon the body. He should know what takes place under his hands as he applies superficial or deep stroking, kneading, or friction massage. He should be able to correlate technical skill and physiological knowledge, thus adding greatly to his satisfaction and enabling him to give effective service to his patients.

Even though the physician writes his hydrotherapy and massage prescription carefully, it is still necessary for the therapist to exercise judgment in its administration, judgment based upon his experience and his knowledge of physiological principles. It may be necessary at times to vary technique somewhat as he observes the patient's physiological and psychological response to the prescribed procedure. The ability to observe and think makes the difference between a mere technician and a well-trained therapist. Experience is an excellent teacher to those who have the essential training.

Because of the importance of knowledge of the physical properties of water and the physiological effects of hydrotherapy and massage to the well-qualified nurse or physical therapist, two chapters on basic physics and physiology have been included in this volume, one on hydrotherapy and the other on massage. It is suggested that these chapters be studied before the training in technique is begun.

Then as each new procedure is introduced and practiced in the laboratory, an endeavor should be made to observe as many of the physiological effects as possible. This will sharpen the student's ability to observe and will add greatly to the value of the course in hydrotherapy and massage.

It is a rewarding experience for one to watch his patient obtain relief from discouragement and pain, and in many cases recover from disease, as a result of the treatment given him.

CONTENTS

SECTION I

HYDROTHERAPY

◇ ◇ ‖ ◇

THE RATIONALE
OF HYDROTHERAPY

INTRODUCTION

The healthy human body maintains a normal uniform physiological stability within and among its parts, a condition known as homeostasis. In order to preserve this homeostatic condition the body must continually make physiological adjustments to environmental influences. Various environmental factors influence physiological processes within the human body. These include seasonal changes, temperature, atmospheric pressure, rainfall, sunlight, the various radiations, clothing, food and water supply, and social conditions.

Mills[1] has stated that the ease with which heat can be lost from the body has a definite effect on various bodily functions, such as growth and reproduction, the production of antibodies, resistance to infection, energy metabolism, and even mental activity.

In hydrotherapy the environment of the body is changed by means of water at varying temperatures and applied by various mechanical means. In general, the physiological responses are in direct proportion to the extent of the environmental changes. If a patient or an experimental subject is placed in a water bath at 97° F., there is minimal physiologic response. In fact, such a bath has a sedative effect by its lack of stimulation of physiological processes. On the other hand, if we place the same subject in a water bath at 110° F., marked physiological changes are immediately apparent. The skin becomes flushed, the pulse rate increases, the temperature rises, metabolism is accelerated, the blood becomes more alkaline, and the white blood cells increase in number. In some subjects there is marked nervous excitement. In twenty minutes the body temperature may reach 104° to 105° F. and the pulse rate as much as 160 beats per minute. Fortunately, water is an exceedingly versatile therapeutic agent, so that the physiological response can be varied at will by changing the temperature and the mechanical impact. It is obvious that real measurable physiological changes can be produced by means of hydrotherapeutic procedures. This is doubtless the reason that hydrotherapy, although one of the oldest therapeutic agents, is still recognized as important by those who are familiar with its application.

DEFINITION

Hydrotherapy may be defined as the use of water in any of its three forms, solid, liquid, or vapor, internally or externally, in the treatment of disease or trauma.

PROPERTIES OF WATER

Water has certain unique properties which render it a valuable therapeutic agent. In the first place, it is readily accessible and may be applied with relatively simple and inexpensive equipment. It possesses the ability to absorb and communicate large quantities of heat. Water is taken as the standard and has a specific heat of 1; i.e., it takes 1 calorie of heat to raise 1 gram of water 1° C. This is a relatively high specific heat as compared to a number of other common substances. Water is also a good conductor of heat. These properties compared with other substances are shown in the accompanying table:

	Specific Heat	Specific Heat Conductivity
Water	1.0	1.0
Alcohol	.59	.33
Glycerin	.57	.50
Paraffin	.69	.45
Air	.23	.043
Mercury	.033	13.0

When the state of water is changed from fluid to vapor, about 540 calories of heat are required for each gram of water vaporized. This is known as the latent heat of vaporization of water, which is defined as the heat required to vaporize one gram of it at a constant temperature. Because of this, the evaporation of water or perspiration from the skin surface has a pronounced cooling effect proportional to the rate of evaporation. When water vapor or steam changes back to liquid, about 540 calories of heat are liberated. This is illustrated by the severe burns which are produced when live steam comes into contact with the skin and condenses on it. When water changes its state from liquid to solid, it loses about eighty calories of heat per gram. Conversely, eighty calories of heat are required to melt a gram of ice. This is known as the latent heat of fusion. For this reason ice is an effective cooling and refrigerating agent.

The fact that water exists in three states, solid, liquid, and gas, within a relatively narrow range of temperature, greatly enhances its therapeutic versatility. As ice, it is effective as a cooling agent. With short application it is stimulating, but with long application it is depressing to physiological processes. In the liquid state water may be applied by packs, immersion baths, sprays, and douches at any desired temperature and pressure. As a vapor, it may be employed in vapor or steam baths and by inhalation. Applied in these different forms and by these various techniques, water lends itself to a wide range of therapeutic uses.

The density of water, being near that of the human body, produces a buoyant effect upon immersion equal to the weight of the water displaced. This is of much value in the neuromuscular reeducation of paralyzed muscles. A partially paralyzed muscle or group of muscles previously unable to move a heavy limb, may, with the assistance of the buoyancy effect of water, be able to do so. Upon immersion of the body in water, hydrostatic pressure is exerted on the body surface. This has the effect of increasing venous and lymph flow from the periphery and of increasing the urine output.

The terms "hot" and "cold" are related to the body temperature; ranges above the body temperature are warm or hot. Below body temperature they are cool or cold. The following table taken from Abbott et al[2] will help clarify what is meant by degrees of hot and cold.

Very hot	104° F. and above
Hot	100° to 104° F.
Warm (neutral 94° to 97°)	92° to 100° F.
Tepid	80° to 92° F.
Cool	70° to 80° F.
Cold	55° to 70° F.
Very cold	32° to 55° F.

PHYSIOLOGICAL EFFECTS

Physiological changes produced in the body by hydrotherapeutic procedures may be classified as thermal, mechanical, and chemical. Thermal effects are produced by the application of water at temperatures above or below that of the body. The greater the variation, either above or below the temperature of the body, the greater the physiological effect produced, other factors being equal. The mechanical effects of water upon the body are produced by the impact of the water upon the skin surface in whirlpools, sprays, douches, and frictions. The chemical effects of water are produced when it is taken by mouth or when it is used as an irrigation of some body cavity, such as the large bowel.

Of these three effects, the thermal is by far the most important.

According to the kinetic theory, heat is defined as the kinetic energy of moving particles. This means that in a heated object or substance its molecules are moving at an accelerated rate. In the case of water when it is heated, molecules escape from its surface, and we say that it is evaporating.

Heat may be transferred from one object or substance to another or generated in a substance or tissue by one of the following methods: (1) conduction, (2) convection, or (3) conversion. In conduction, heat is transferred by contact of one heated object or substance with another. This is the manner in which heat is transferred to the body in hydrotherapy. In convection, heat is transferred by moving currents of heated liquids or gases, as in the hot-air furnace or the automobile radiator. In conversion, heat is generated in a substance or tissue by the passage through it of some form of energy; e.g., the heating of a wire or filament by electricity or the heating of body tissue by diathermy or ultrasound. As indicated above, the heating and cooling effects of water are produced by conduction. The contact of water with the body is accomplished by means of packs, immersion baths, sprays, douches, and vapor baths, and by drinking water.

In the therapeutic use of water, it is essential that a means of measuring temperature be found. This is accomplished by various types of thermometers employing either Fahrenheit or Centigrade scale. The corresponding points on these two scales are shown in the table below.

Fahrenheit		Centigrade
212°	Boiling Point of Water	100°
98.6°	Human Body Temperature	37°
+32°	Freezing Point of Water	0°

Conversion from one scale to the other:

(1) C. to F. — Multiply by ⅝ and add 32.
Example: (⅝ × 37) + 32 equals 98.6.

(2) F. to C. — Subtract 32 and multiply by ⅝.
Example: (98.6 — 32) × ⅝ equals 37.

LOCAL EFFECTS OF HEAT

The conductive heat of hydrotherapy does not penetrate deeply beneath the skin surface and is confined largely to the skin and subcutaneous tissues. A recent study by Abrahamson et al[3] indicates that a long, intense application of moist heat penetrates as much as 3.4 centimeters to reach superficial layers of muscle. In these tissues, however, definite physiological responses occur. This is due to the fact that local heat is rapidly dissipated by the increased blood flow mentioned below. The most obvious change is local redness caused by vasodilatation which, according to Wakim et al[4], may be produced by local axon reflexes initiated by stimulation of skin receptors. Landis[5] studied capillary pressure in local heated areas and demonstrated marked increases in pressure in both the arterial and the venous limbs of the capillary. Goldschmidt and Light[6] found that local heating of the forearm and hand caused such a marked increase in blood flow that venous blood returning from the hand was indistinguishable from arterial blood as to oxygen content.

In Abrahamson's[3] recent study the application of "wet heat" to the forearm for a period of twenty to thirty minutes at a temperature of 113° F. increased the rate of blood flow twofold, the increase persisting approximately one hour after the termination of the heating procedure. He and his associates also demonstrated a marked increase in the oxygen content of venous blood, but it was not indistinguishable from arterial blood as to oxygen content.

Krusen, Wakim, *et al*[7], demonstrated that the application of Kenny packs to all four extremities produced significant increases in local blood flow as measured by the occlusion plethysmograph. There is an increase in local tissue metabolism according to Wakim *et al*[8], and the metabolites so produced aid in the local vasodilatation by direct chemical effect. According to van't Hoff's law the velocity of simple chemical reactions increases two to three times for each rise of 10° C.

There is also an increased migration of leukocytes through vessel walls in local heated areas. Muscles in the area under the influence of hydrotherapeutic heat are relaxed, as demonstrated by Benson[9]. Local sweating and local analgesia are produced by moist heat.

LOCAL EFFECTS OF COLD

Because of the fact that the local application of cold produces vasoconstriction, there is no influx of fresh warm blood to the part. As a result, cold penetrates deeply into the tissues from the surface. Bierman[10] made the following comparison of the effects of heat and cold on the temperatures of the skin, subcutaneous tissues, and muscle tissue of the calf.

	Hot-Water Bag		Ice Bag	
	Before	*After*	*Before*	*After*
Skin	90° F.	110° (30 min.)	84°	43° (15 min.)
Subcutaneous tissue	91.5° F.	105.5° (40 min.)	94°	70° (60 min.)
Muscle	94.2° F.	99.5° (50 min.)	98°	79° (120 min.)

In addition to vasoconstriction, the local application of cold causes a slowing of the local circulation, less leukocytic migration through capillary walls, and a decrease in tissue metabolism. An interesting effect of local cold application is a numbing, analgesic, or anesthetic effect. This has been used for the relief of certain types of acute pain, such as: (1) acute joint pain, (2) pain of acute bursitis, (3) sprains and other acute trauma. It has been employed in refrigeration anesthesia for the amputation of gangrenous lower extremities in arteriosclerosis obliterans. In refrigeration anesthesia for amputation of an extremity, the limb is cooled with ice bags for thirty minutes. The leg is then elevated and allowed to blanch. A tourniquet is applied just above the level of amputation. A rubber sheet is placed under the extremity, extending from three or four inches above the tourniquet to the feet. Ice is now packed around the extremity. Depending on the level of amputation, ice is left in place from one to two and one-half hours before surgery is started. The advantages of this method are: (1) ease and speed of surgery; (2) absence of pain before, during, and after surgery; (3) absence of shock; (4) little disturbance of eating and other habits; (5) safety in poor-risk patients. See Carter and Moor[11]. Local cold has also been used in the treatment of burns, immersion foot, and frostbite.

What promises to be a major advance in the treatment of burns is the simple application of cold water. Although used for many years in folk medicine, it was first described in medical literature by Rose[12] in 1936. He found that the early application of cold water to burns in human patients caused immediate relief of pain, limited tissue damage, and reduced the mortality from 14 percent in a group of 130 control cases to 8 percent in fifty-two treated cases. Ofeigsson[13], Zitowitz and Hardy[14], and Reynolds, et al[15] in experiments on rats and dogs demonstrated that immediate application of cold water to burned areas decreased tissue damage, hastened healing, and greatly lowered mortality. The optimal temperature range was found to be from 65° to 70° F.

Shulman[16] recently reported the immediate local application of ice water (40° to 55° F.) in a series of 150 patients with thermal burns over less than 20 percent of the body surface. In every instance pain was relieved immediately and redness and blistering reduced. The duration of immersion ranged from thirty minutes to five hours. The immersion was continued until the pain did not recur when the treatment was interrupted.

Information concerning early application of cold water in the treatment of burns should be widely disseminated, so that it can be applied immediately after the injury occurs. The earlier cold water is applied, the less will be the severity of the lesion.

REFLEX OR CONSENSUAL EFFECTS

A sufficiently intense local application of heat or cold to the skin surface not only affects the immediate skin area, but exerts also remote reflex or consensual effects elsewhere in the body through the nervous system. For example, an ice bag applied over the precordial area slows the heart rate and increases its force. A fomentation applied to the skin of the abdomen causes diminished intestinal activity, decreased intestinal blood flow, and decreased gastric acid secretion.

The effects described above are mediated through a reflex arc made up of an afferent nerve fiber from the skin surface which carries the stimulus to the spinal cord through the posterior nerve root. Here it is communicated through synapses to an efferent autonomic fiber which leaves the cord with an anterior spinal nerve root from which it branches by a white ramus communicans to enter an autonomic ganglion. Within the ganglion the stimulus passes through another synapse and proceeds to the organ supplied, or returns by way of a gray ramus communicans to the spinal nerve trunk and travels with it to their mutual destination. In general the skin area over an organ is in reflex relationship to it, although there are exceptions to this rule which will be mentioned later. These relationships may be seen in the diagram of the reflex arc. (See next page.)

Reflex or consensual effects may be classified under three headings: (1) vasomotor or circulatory; (2) visceromotor or muscular; and (3) secretory or glandular. All these effects are illus-

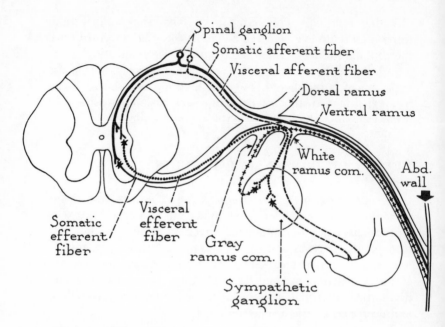

trated in a reflex effect on the gastrointestinal tract mentioned in a preceding paragraph.

A considerable amount of study has been done by many investigators, some of it in recent years, on the reflex relationships of skin and viscera.

Reflex effects are based anatomically on the segmental relationships of the skin and viscera. The pioneer work on these relationships was done independently by Head[17] and Mackenzie[18] in their monumental studies on referred pain. They demonstrated that painful impulses from an insensitive diseased viscus produces referred pain in the skin area receiving sensory innervation from the same segment of the spinal cord. Head found that when a painful stimulus occurred in an area of low sensitivity (a viscus) which is in reflex relationship with an area of high sensitivity (the skin), pain is felt in the latter area. The following table shows these viscerocutaneous relationships.

SEGMENTAL RELATIONSHIPS OF SKIN AND VISCERA

Organs	Segments
Heart and aorta	Dorsal 1-4
Lungs	Dorsal 1-7 (commonly 2-5)
Stomach	Dorsal 7-9
Intestines	Dorsal 9-11
Liver and gall bladder	Dorsal 3, 6-9
Kidneys	Dorsal 10 to Lumbar 1
Testes	Dorsal 10
Bladder Mucosa	Sacral 3-4
Bladder Muscle	Dorsal 11 to Lumbar 1
Uterus, upper portion	Dorsal 11, 12
Uterus, lower portion	Sacral 3-4

Poulton[19] demonstrated in 1928 that the function of the esophagus could be influenced by irritation of the skin over the sternum. Freude and Ruhmann[20] and Ruhmann[21] reported that cold applied to the epigastrium causes lessening of tone of the stomach with complete quieting of the pylorus. Heat at 50° C. to the epigastrium produced increased tone in a relaxed stomach and decreased tone in a contracted stomach. These stimuli were found to be specific for the skin area over the stomach.

Bing and Tobiassen[22] demonstrated reflex relationships between the skin of the abdominal wall and the colon. Bing[23] also demonstrated a reflex relationship between the lungs and the skin of the chest wall. Grossmann[24] claimed that reflex pathways from viscera to skin can be traversed also from skin to viscera. Stewart[25], Hewlett[26], and Briscoe[27] all observed changes in blood flow in the opposite hand and arm when one hand and arm were placed in hot or cold water. Kuntz[28] in his discussion of cutaneovisceral reflexes said, "In view of the facility with which cutaneous stimulation elicits reflex visceral reactions, particularly vasomotor changes and changes in the tonic state of the visceral musculature, it must be apparent that many visceral disorders, particularly disorders of the gastrointestinal canal, may be influenced beneficially by appropriate stimulation of the corresponding cutaneous area."

Dittmar[29] recently presented a review of the evidence, mostly in the German literature, for the view that visceral function can be influenced reflexly by stimulation of segmentally related skin areas. He first observed clinically that pain of gastric origin could be eliminated by the injection of procain into the related reflex area, T7-8. This led to further investigation by means of experiments on animals. In his own laboratory he demonstrated in anesthetized dogs and rabbits that stimulation of the reflex area for the stomach, T7-8, by mechanical means, by faradic stimulation, or by ultrasound, caused cessation of motor activity.

Fischer and Solomon[30] wrote, "Externally applied heat not only decreases intestinal blood flow, but also diminishes intestinal motility and decreases acid secretion in the stomach, while cold has the opposite effect."

"This must be a reflex action, since warming or cooling the stomach directly by oral administration of hot liquid or ice water increases or decreases respectively gastric motility and acid secretion as is to be expected from a direct temperature effect on the stomach."

Gibbon and Landis[31] found that when the hands and forearms of a normal human subject are immersed in water at 112° to 115° F., the temperature of the toes rises rapidly from about 70° F. to the same temperature as the forehead, about 90° F. This is a striking example of a more complex reflex effect which is bound up with the temperature control of the body. The Gibbon-Landis procedure is employed as a diagnostic test in occlusive diseases of the peripheral arteries. (See next page.)

In our own laboratory we have demonstrated some striking general reflex circulatory responses to various skin stimuli. An understanding of these is of considerable importance to the hydrotherapist. In these experiments the forearm of the experimental subject was placed in a volume-measuring chamber, a plethysmograph, with a recording system set up to write on a

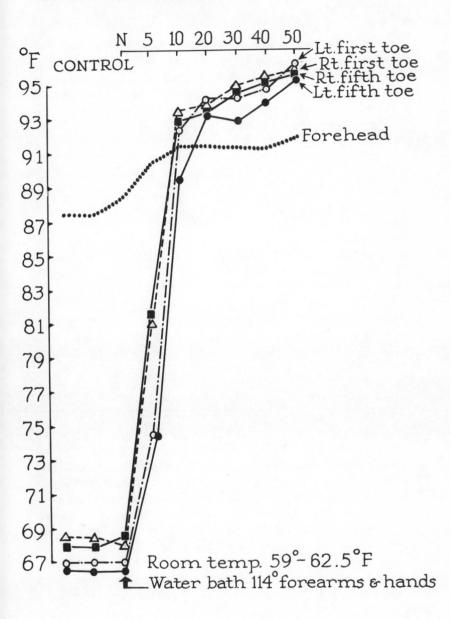

revolving kymograph. By application of infrared heat to the lower extremities, maximal peripheral vasodilatation was produced as indicated by the increase in recorded arm volume. Figure 3 shows the effect of various stimuli on arm volume while the heat was still applied to the body. These experiments demonstrate the very close relationship between the environment and the circulatory status in the body. (Dail and Moor[32].)

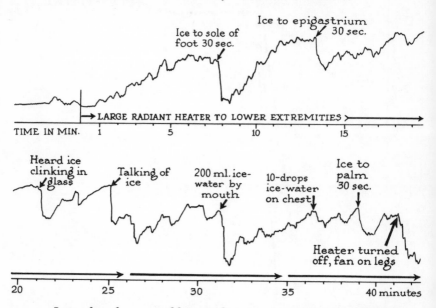

It is, therefore, possible to influence visceral function by the application of thermal stimuli, hot or cold, to skin areas reflexly related to the viscera. As already indicated, the internal organs are usually reflexly related to the overlying skin, but there are a number of more remote areas related to some organs, although the nervous pathways may be difficult to trace. The figure on page 15 shows the location of reflex areas for various viscera and certain other tissues.

The direct local effects of heat and cold have already been described. It has been taught in the past that effects in reflexly

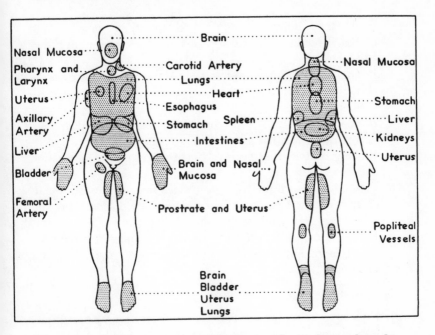

related organs or tissues were the same as those observed in the local reflex skin area. This has not always been found to be the case in studies that have been made. The best example of the contrary effect is the effect of heat to the abdominal skin on the gastrointestinal tract which has already been mentioned. Here prolonged heat to the abdomen decreases instead of increasing intestinal blood flow, diminishes intestinal motility, and decreases instead of increasing acid secretion in the stomach. Prolonged cold, on the other hand, has opposite effects. The following reflex effects have either been verified by experimental study or are obvious from clinical observation.

Reflex effects of prolonged heat

1. Prolonged heat to one extremity causes vasodilatation in the contralateral extremity.
2. Prolonged heat to the abdominal wall causes decreased intes-

tinal blood flow and diminished intestinal motility, and decreases secretion of acid in the stomach, according to Fisher and Solomon[30].

3. Prolonged heat to the pelvis relaxes the musculature of the pelvic organs, dilates the blood vessels, and increases menstrual flow.

4. Prolonged heat to the precordium increases the heart rate, decreases its force, and lowers blood pressure.

5. Prolonged moist heat to the chest promotes ease of respiration and expectoration.

6. Prolonged heat to the trunk, such as a hot trunk pack, apparently relaxes the ureters or bile ducts, as the case may be, and relieves renal or gallbladder colic.

7. Prolonged moist heat to the area over the kidneys in the back and over the lower abdomen in front increases the production of urine.

Reflex effects of prolonged cold

1. Prolonged cold over the trunk of an artery produces contraction of the artery and its branches.

2. Prolonged cold to the skin over the nose, the back of the neck, and the hands causes contraction of the blood vessels of the nasal mucosa. See Spiesman and Arnold[33].

3. An ice bag applied to the precordium slows the heart rate and increases its stroke volume.

4. Prolonged cold to skin of the abdomen causes increased intestinal blood flow, increased intestinal motility, and increased acid secretion in the stomach, according to Fischer and Solomon[30].

5. Cold to the pelvic area, e.g., a cold sitz bath, stimulates the muscles of pelvic organs; useful in subinvolution of the uterus.

6. An ice pack over the thyroid gland contracts its blood vessels and decreases its function.

7. Prolonged cold to the hands and the skin of the scalp causes contraction of blood vessels of the brain.

8. Prolonged cold over acutely inflamed joints or bursae causes

vasoconstriction and relief of pain, and hastens recovery.
9. Prolonged cold in the form of the ice pack or cold immersion in acute trauma such as contusions and sprains causes vaso-constriction and lessens pain, swelling, and hemorrhage into the tissues. These effects are probably only partially reflex.

Reflex effects of short cold

1. In a warm environment when the vessels of the skin are dilated a local application of intense cold as brief as 30 seconds will cause a general peripheral vasoconstriction. See figure on page 14.
2. A very brief cold application to the face, hands, and head causes an increase in mental alertness and activity.
3. Very short cold applications to the precordial area cause an increase in the heart's rate and stroke volume.
4. It is probably true, although it lacks experimental verification, that short intense cold stimuli, such as the percussion douche, applied to the reflex area of one of the internal organs will increase the functional activity of the organ. The author has seen clinical evidence that this is true of the liver.
5. Short cold applications to the chest, with friction or percussion effects, first increase respiratory rate, but then induce a slower, deeper respiration.

Reflex effects by alternating hot and cold procedures

1. Short alternating heat and cold have a marked stimulating effect on reflexly related tissues and organs. An example of this is the contrast bath, the effects of which have been studied by Wakim[34] and will be described later. There can be little doubt that alternating heat and cold, or the contrast bath, is among the most potent procedures that exist in hydro-therapy treatments.

HYDROSTATIC EFFECT

When a large area of the body or the whole body surface is exposed to heat, a general dilatation of the blood vessels of the skin takes place. This is the body's method of eliminating heat. In this process, however, a large quantity of blood has been shifted from the interior of the body to the skin. This results in a considerable depletion of blood volume from the interior of the body. Fischer and Solomon[30] say, "It has been experimentally proven that when a subject is exposed acutely to a cold environment considerable blood is shifted from the limbs to the lungs, while when exposed to a warm environment a shift in the opposite direction occurs."

This shifting of fluid from one part of the body to another has been known in hydrotherapy as a hydrostatic effect. It can be used clinically in the treatment of conditions in which it is suspected that there is a locally congested area which is giving rise to symptoms. One example is the so-called congestive headache; another is the congested condition of the nose and accessory sinuses in the common cold; and a third, the pulmonary congestion in the early stages of lobar pneumonia. Derivation, or dilatation of the blood vessels of the skin, is usually effective in relieving the congested condition.

Local effects of alternating heat and cold

Local alternating heat and cold, also called contrast, produce marked stimulation of local circulation. Wakim et al[34] demonstrated that a thirty-minute contrast bath produced a 95 percent increase in local blood flow when the lower extremities alone were immersed. When all four extremities were immersed simultaneously, there was a 100 percent increase in blood flow in the upper extremities and a 70 percent increase in the lower extremities.

Study has been given to the optimal immersion times in the contrast bath. Woodmansey et al[35] of England found six-minute immersion periods in hot water and four minutes in cold water to be optimal for British subjects. Krusen[36] found immersion for four minutes in hot water and for one minute in cold to be optimal. The writer has used hot-water immersion for three minutes and cold-water immersion for thirty to sixty seconds for a total of thirty minutes with satisfactory results in clinical practice. The cold immersion needs only to be long enough to produce vasoconstriction and this can be shown to occur in as little as twenty seconds. Because of its marked stimulation of local blood flow, the contrast bath is an exceedingly useful hydrotherapeutic procedure.

GENERAL EFFECTS OF HEAT

Of greatest importance to the hydrotherapist are the mechanisms of heat loss. Seventy percent of heat loss at ordinary room temperatures is via the skin by radiation, convection, and conduction; 27 percent by evaporation from the skin and lungs; 2 percent by warming of the inspired air; and 1 percent by the excreta. As the environmental temperature rises and approaches that of the body (93° to 95° F.) radiation, convection, and conduction cease to be effective, and heat loss from the skin is accomplished entirely by evaporation of perspiration. Heat loss from the skin is modified by the clothing, by environmental temperature, and by the humidity of the environmental air. When the humidity of the air is high, heat elimination by evaporation is impaired and, with complete saturation of the air, is prevented; actual fever then results.

General applications of heat by means of full hot packs, immersion baths, or hot vapor baths produce definite physiological responses. These responses are an attempt at heat elimination to prevent a rise in the body temperature. The peripheral blood vessels dilate to promote loss of heat by radiation, convection, conduction, and evaporation from the skin. There is a marked increase in the rate of blood flow which, according to Bierman[37], may be as much as 400 percent. The pulse rate increases about ten beats per minute per degree Fahrenheit rise in temperature, according to Bazett[38]. However, in a study of 125 artificial-fever treatments given in a saturated atmosphere at 110°, we found an average increase in pulse rate of 6 per degree Fahrenheit rise in temperature (Moor[39]). General applications of moist heat above 104° F. not only increase the heart rate but decrease the stroke volume. The systolic blood pressure usually rises initially upon general exposure to moist heat but subsequently falls to normal or lower. The diastolic blood pressure falls, thus increasing the pulse pressure.

General applications of moist heat produce an increase in the respiratory rate of five or six respirations per degree Fahrenheit rise in temperature. There is a tendency to hyperventilation, especially when the temperature rise is rapid, thereby eliminating an excess of carbon dioxide in the expired air with a resulting increase in the pH of the blood and alkalosis. With prolonged applications of heat, this may cause actual tetany with carpopedal spasm, oppression in the chest, and excitement. One effective remedy for alkalosis and tetany is to hold the breath and allow an accummulation of carbon dioxide to occur in the blood.

General applications of moist heat cause quantitative changes in the cells of the blood. The leukocytes are increased, as demonstrated by Krusen[40], who recorded the white blood count before and after artificial fever of 104° to 107.8° F. The average count before fever was 7,125 cells per cu. mm. of blood and 11,270 cells per cu. mm. after. There was a relative increase in the neutrophils.

Hargraves and Doan[41] found the peak leukocytosis, several hours after completion of the fever, approximately 40,000 white blood cells per cu. mm. of blood. The increase in the white blood cells following several hours of artificial fever is greater than would occur after a short hot bath, but the latter is of the same nature. It is interesting to note that McCutcheon[42] observed an increase in the movements of white blood cells with a rise in body temperature to 104° F., where they were maximal. From these changes in the white blood cells it appears that general applications of heat, especially when prolonged, mobilize the body's defenses against disease.

Under the influence of a general application of moist heat there is a shift of fluid from the tissues to the blood stream thus increasing blood volume and causing a slight dilution of the blood with a relative decrease in the number of red cells per cubic millimeter. With long-continued heating, as in fever therapy of several hours duration, concentration occurs with a relative increase in the number of cells per cubic millimeter.

General applications of moist heat cause profuse sweating with loss of water, salt, and small amounts of urea, uric acid, creatinine, phosphates, sulfates, and lactic acid. Under ordinary conditions of health, the skin is not an important excreter of nitrogenous wastes (urea, uric acid, and creatinine). When kidney function is impaired, however, the skin may excrete an increased quantity of urea. Pemberton, Cajori, and Crouter[43] found increased excretion of nitrogen in the sweat of patients suffering from nephritis. Increased excretion in the sweat coincided with increased blood urea nitrogen.

Pemberton[44] was of the opinion that the production of sweating by means of hot moist packs was of definite value in the treatment of nephritis. He said further that clinicians of his acquaintance shared his opinion. Plaggemeyer and Marshall[45], although they found the concentration of urea in the sweat three to ten times that in the blood, and although they had studied no cases of nephritis, did not believe that sweating would be of value in the treatment of nephritis with nitrogen retention. The writer has used the full blanket pack in the treatment of nephritis with nitrogen retention. If fluid intake is maintained so that the nitrogenous waste remaining in the blood is not concentrated, hydrotherapy is of value.

GENERAL APPLICATIONS OF COLD

Prolonged exposure of the body to cold in an air-conditioned room or an immersion bath exerts the intrinsic effect of cold, which is depression of physiological function. The general metabolism is decreased, the temperature falls, the heart rate is decreased, the circulation is slower, the respiratory rate is decreased, cutaneous sensation is depressed, the muscles are sluggish and clumsy, digestion is retarded, and the subject becomes stuporous.

3—M.H.M.

The temperature-reducing effect of the prolonged cold immersion bath is used in the treatment of heat hyperpyrexia or "sunstroke." However, Baruch[46] has called attention to the fact that the mortality rate in heat hyperpyrexia is much lower when the body is douched with water at 60° to 70° F. accompanied by friction. Before the introduction of chloramphenicol (antibiotic), the Brand bath, a cold immersion bath, was formerly used successfully in the treatment of typhoid fever.

Some years ago, Fay[47] introduced the use of general refrigeration by means of ice packs or air conditioning to produce hypothermia in the experimental treatment of severe pain and to retard the growth of cancer. It was reported to accomplish both these results. Hypothermia has been reported to be useful in the treatment of morphine addiction and schizophrenia.

Recently, general hypothermia has been used in connection with open heart surgery. Zinn and Warnock[48] have recently described the procedure. The patient is first sedated with meperidine, scopolamine, and a mild tranquilizer. Anesthesia is induced with ether and nitrous oxide. The patient is transferred to a shallow tub containing finely crushed ice covered with a single sheet blanket. He is covered with a second sheet blanket and a one- to two-inch layer of ice from the neck down. In fifty to ninety minutes the patient's temperature has dropped to 88° to 91° F. He is then shifted to the operating table, and by the time the operation starts, his temperature, taken by rectal thermocouple, is 79° to 88° F. It is possible for the patient to tolerate circulatory occlusion for fifteen minutes at this temperature while cardiac surgery is in progress.

USE OF COLD IN SPASTICITY

Recently both local and general applications of cold have been employed in the symptomatic treatment of the spasticity of upper motor neuron lesions. Levine et al[49] demonstrated an actual increase in spasticity in response to heat. However, upon the application of wet cold at 50° F. they observed a decrease in spasticity. This was applied, in cases of multiple sclerosis, locally and by immersion to the waist. Watson[50] in a careful study in cases of multiple sclerosis found that exposure to cold air at 40° F., immersion in cold water at 70° to 80°, or wrapping in a cold wet blanket produced a decrease in spasticity as well as improvement in impaired vision, dysarthria, impaired sensation, depressed mood, ophthalmoplegia, and ataxic spastic paraparesis.

Mead (unpublished paper) uses local wet cold packs in the spasticity of multiple sclerosis, cerebrovascular accidents, and postoperative spasticity. Boynton et al[51] also observed favorable results from immersion of spastic multiple sclerosis patients in water at 80° F. Physical therapists Basset and Lake [52] and Viel[53] also reported relaxation of spastic muscles in response to cold applications.

The techniques employed in the application of cold in spastic cases have varied greatly as indicated above. It appears that both local and general applications are effective in relief of spasticity. No standard technique has yet been developed. Procedures have varied from repeated three-second local exposures at 35° to 40° F. to twenty minutes general exposures at 70° to 80° F.

The mode of action of cold in producing relaxation of spasticity is unknown. The work of Zausmer[54] may furnish a clue. He observed that a decrease in human skin temperature caused a decrease in local motor excitability. Mead[55] speculated that "cold anesthesia of peripheral sensory end organs changes the balance of the algebraic sum of facilitatory-inhibitory influences playing on the anterior horn cell in favor of inhibition."

REACTION

An important use of general cold applications in hydrotherapy is the production of the phenomenon known as *reaction*. This is the response of the body to a brief hot or cold stimulus. Really, to appreciate fully this interesting physiological response, one must experience it himself. Reaction to cold is produced by a brief, vigorous application of cold water. This may be accomplished by means of the cold mitten friction, the cold wet sheet rub, the cold spray, the percussion douche, or the immersion bath. The reaction is enhanced by mechanical stimuli such as friction or the pressure impact of water in the spray or douche. The treatment must be given with vigor and speed. Thorough drying and vigorous friction are essential. The environmental temperature should be at least 72° F. Meticulous attention to detail is the secret of good hydrotherapy.

What happens in this phenomenon of reaction? The heat regulating mechanism of the body endeavors to maintain thermal and circulatory equilibrium against the cold stimulus. We, therefore, have three phases in reaction: (1) the thermic phase, (2) the circulatory phase, and (3) the nervous phase. The most obvious phase is the circulatory phase in which, through the autonomic nervous system, a primary cutaneous vasoconstriction is produced followed very quickly by vasodilatation manifested by a warm feeling, tingling, and a rosy skin. Other circulatory responses occurring during reaction to cold are a slowing of the heart rate and a slight rise in the blood pressure. The thermic phase of the reaction is increased heat production to combat the cold stimulus. There is also reflex nervous stimulation with increased muscle tone and a general feeling of increased vigor and well-being.

An incomplete reaction is undesirable and is manifested by cyanosis of the skin, chilliness and shivering, cold hands and feet, and fullness in the head. These symptoms can be combated by an application of heat to a part or all of the body. Such incomplete reactions are likely to occur in persons of low vitality such as the very young or the very old and those suffering from or convalescing from chronic debilitating disease. Fatigue also tends to interfere with reaction. Such persons will react better after a preliminary heating procedure. It is well to remember that all patients react better following preliminary heat or exercise.

The reaction to heat is atonic and relaxing. It is of considerable value for its sedative effect. Occasional patients may be stimulated by it.

References

1. Mills, C. A.: *Medical Climatology*. Springfield, Charles C. Thomas, 1939.
2. Abbott, G. K.; Moor, F. B.; and Nelson, K. J.: *Physical Therapy in Nursing Care*. Washington, D.C., Review and Herald Publishing Association, 1941.
3. Abrahamson, D. I.; Mitchell, R. E.; Turk, S.; Bell, Y; and Zayas, A. M.: "Changes in Blood Flow, Oxygen Uptake and Tissue Temperatures Produced by Topical Applications of Wet Heat." *Arch. Phys. Med. and Rehab.* 42:305 (May), 1961.
4. Wakim, K. G.: "The Physiological Effects of Heat." *J.A.M.A.* 138:109 (Dec. 11), 1948.
5. Landis, E. M.: "Micro-Injection Studies of Capillary Blood Pressure in Human Skin." *Heart* 15:209 (May), 1930.
6. Goldschmidt, S.; and Light, A. B.: "The Effect of Local Temperature Upon Peripheral Circulation and Metabolism of Tissues as Revealed by Gaseous Content of Venous Blood." *Am. J. Physiol.* 73:146, 1925.
7. Krusen, E. M.; Wakim, K. G.; Leden, U. M.; Martin, G. M.; and Elkins, E. C.: "Effect of Hot Packs on the Peripheral Circulation." *Arch. Phys. Med. and Rehab.* 31:145 (March), 1950.
8. Wakim, K. G.; Wise, C .S.; and Moor, F. B.: "Basic Fundamentals and Clinical Applications for Heat and Cold." *Med. Arts and Sc.* 13:126 (No. 3), 1959.
9. Benson, S.: "Volume Changes in Organs Induced by the Local Application of External Heat and Cold and by Diathermy." *Arch. Phys. Ther.* 15:133 (Feb.), 1934.
10. Bierman, W.; and Licht, S.: *Physical Medicine in General Practice*. New York, Paul B. Haeber, Inc., 1952.
11. Carter, R.; and Moor, F. B.: "Refrigeration Anesthesia." *Arch. Phys. Med.* 28:712 (Nov.), 1947.
12. Rose, H. W.: "Initial Cold Water Treatment of Burns." *Northwest Med.* 35:267 (June), 1936.
13. Ofeigsson, O. J.: "First Aid Treatment of Scalds and Burns by Water Cooling." *Postgrad. Med.* 30:330 (Oct.), 1961.
14. Zitowitz, I.; and Hardy, J. D.: "Influence of Cold Exposure on Thermal Burns in the Rat." *J. Appl. Physiol.* 12:147 (Jan.), 1958.
15. Reynolds, L. E.; Brown, C. R.; and Price, P. B.: "Effects of Local Chilling in the Treatment of Burns." *S. Forum* 6:85-87, 1955.
16. Shulman, A. G.: "Ice Water in the Primary Treatment of Burns." *J.A.M.A.* 173:1916 (Aug. 27), 1960.
17. Head, H.: "On Disturbances of Sensation With Especial Reference to the Pain of Visceral Disease." *Brain* 16:1, 1893.

18. Mackenzie, J.: "Associated Pain of Visceral Disease." *Med. Chronicle* 16:295 (Aug.), 1892.
19. Poulton, E. P.: "An Experimental Study of Certain Visceral Sensations." *Lancet* 215:1223, also *Lancet* 215:1277, 1928.
20. Freude, E.; and Ruhmann, W.: "Über Viscerale Reflexe auf locale thermische Hautreize." *Ztschr. f. d. ges. exper. Med.* 52:769, 1927.
21. Ruhmann, W.: "Reflex Irritability of Abdominal Organs by Local Application of Heat and Cold. Preliminary Report." *Munchen Med. Wchnschr.* 73:401 (March 5), 1926.
22. Bing, H. J.; and Tobiassen, E. S.: "Viscerocutaneous and Cutovisceral Abdominal Reflexes." *Acta Med. Scandinav.* Supp. 78:824, 1936.
23. Bing, H. J.: "Viscerocutaneous and Cutovisceral Thoracic Reflexes." *Acta Med. Scandinav.* 89:57, 1936.
24. Grossmann, W.: "Über reflektorische Beziehungen zwischen Haut und Harnorganen." *Klin. Wchnschr.* 11:1181 (July 9), 1932.
25. Stewart, G. N.: "The Effect of Reflex Vasomotor Excitation on the Blood Flow in the Hand." *Heart* 3:76, 1912.
26. Hewlett, A. W.; Van Zwaluwenburg, J. G.; and Marshall, M.: "The Effect of Some Hydrotherapeutic Procedures on the Blood Flow in the Arm." *Arch. Int. Med.* 8:591 (Nov.), 1911.
27. Briscoe, G.: "Observations on Venous and Capillary Pressures With Special Reference to the 'Raynaud Phenomena.'" *Heart* 7:35, 1918.
28. Kuntz, A.: *Autonomic Nervous System.* Philadelphia, Lea & Febiger, 1945, p. 512.
29. Dittmar, F.: "Viscerocutaneous and Cutivisceral Reflexes and Their Importance for Physical and Neurological Medicine." *Wiener Med. Wchnschr.* 110:840 (Oct.), 1960.
30. Fischer, E.; and Solomon, S.: "Physiological Responses to Heat and Cold." In *Therapeutic Heat,* Edited by Sidney Licht. New Haven, Conn. Pub. Elizabeth Licht. 1958.
31. Gibbon, J. H.; and Landis, E. M.: "Vasodilatation in Lower Extremities in Response to Immersing the Forearms in Warm Water." *J. Clin. Investigation* 11:1019 (Sept.), 1932.
32. Dail, C. W.; and Moor, F. B.: "Effects of Heat, Cold, and Other Stimuli Upon the Human Circulation." *Arch. Phys. Ther.* 19:135 (March), 1938.
33. Spiesman, I. G.; and Arnold, L.: "Host Susceptibility to the Common Cold." *Amer. J. Dig. Dis. and Nutrit.* 4:438, 1937.
34. Engel, J. P.; Wakim, K. G.; Erickson, D. J.; and Krusen, F. H.: "The Effect of Contrast Baths on the Peripheral Circulation of Patients With Rheumatoid Arthritis." *Arch. Phys. Med.* 31:135, 1950.
35. Woodmansey, A.; Collins, D. H.; and Ernst, M. M.: "Vascular Reactions to the Contrast Bath in Health and in Rheumatoid Arthritis." *Lancet* 2:1350 (Dec. 10), 1938.
36. Krusen, F. H.: *Physical Medicine.* Philadelphia, W. B. Saunders Co., 1941.
37. Bierman, W.; and Kissin, M.: "Influence of Hyperpyrexia on the

Velocity of Blood Flow." *Proc. Soc. Exper. Biol. and Med.* 30:527 (Jan.), 1933.

38. Bazett, H. C.: "Studies of the Effects of Baths on Man—I: Relationship Between the Effects Produced and the Temperature of the Bath." *Am. J. Physiol.* 70:412 (Oct.), 1924.

39. Moor, F. B.; and Miller, V. J.: "Acute Effects of a Hot Saturated Atmosphere Upon the Human Temperature, Heart Rate, and Blood Pressure as Influenced by Age." *British J. Phys. Med.* 10:167 (Nov.-Dec.), 1947.

40. Krusen, F. H.: "The Blood Picture Before and After Fever Therapy by Physical Means." *Am. J. Med. Sc.* 193:470 (April), 1937.

41. Hargraves, M. M.; and Doan, C. A.: "The Physiological Response of the Hemopoietic Tissues to Artificially Induced Fever." *Ann. Fever Conf.* 5:51, 1935.

42. McCutcheon, M.: "Studies on the Locomotion of Leukocytes—II: The Effect of Temperature on the Locomotion of Human Neutrophilic Leukocytes in Vitro." *Am. J. Physiol.* 66:125 (Sept. 25), 1923.

43. Pemberton, R.; Cajori, F. A.; and Crouter, C. Y.: "A Note on the Composition of Human Sweat." *Ann. Int. Med.* 2:1243, 1929.

44. Pemberton, R.; Weisenburg, T. H.; Gill, A. B.; and Schamberg, J. F.: "The Influence and Therapeutic Use of External Heat." *J.A.M.A.* 89:1243 (Oct.), 1927.

45. Plaggemeyer, H. W.; and Marshall, E. K.: "A Comparison of the Excretory Power of the Skin With That of the Kidney Through the Study of Human Sweat." *Arch. Int. Med.* 13:159 (Jan.), 1914.

46. Baruch, S.: *An Epitome of Hydrotherapy.* Philadelphia. W. B. Saunders Co., 1920.

47. Fay, T.: "Observations on Prolonged Human Refrigeration." *N.Y. J. Med.* 40:1351 (Sept. 15), 1940.

48. Zinn, W. J.; and Warnock, E. H.: "Safe Hypothermia." *J.A.M.A.* 174:284 (Sept. 17), 1960.

49. Levine, M. G.; Kabat, H.; Knott, M.; and Voss, D. E.: "Relaxation of Spasticity by Physiological Technics." *Arch. Phys. Med. and Rehab.* 35:214 (April), 1954.

50. Watson, C. W.: "Effect of Lowering of Body Temperature on the Symptoms and Signs of Multiple Sclerosis." *New Eng. J. Med.* 261:1253 (Dec. 17), 1959.

51. Boynton, B. L.; Garramone, P. M.; and Buca, J. F.: "Observations on the Effects of Cool Baths for Patients With Multiple Sclerosis." *Phys. Ther. Rev.* 39:297 (May), 1959.

52. Bassett, S. W.; and Lake, B. M.: "Use of Cold Applications in the Management of Spasticity." *Phys. Ther. Rev.* 38:333 (May), 1958.

53. Viel, E.: "Treatment of Spasticity by Exposure to Cold." *Phys. Ther. Rev.* 39:598 (Sept.), 1959.

54. Zausmer, D. M.: "The Effect of Cooling on Muscle Excitability." *Ann. Phys. Med.* 4:144 (Nov.), 1957.

55. Mead, S.: Unpublished report.

◇ ◇ 2 ◇

Technique of Local
THERMAL PROCEDURES

FOMENTATIONS (Fo.)

Definition

A fomentation consists of a local application of moist heat to the body surface. The fomentation cloth is usually made of blanket material, 50 percent wool to retain heat and 50 percent cotton to retain moisture and for greater durability. This material may be purchased by the yard, or, more economically, as ordinary bed blankets (Chatham blankets).

Effects and indications

1. Analgesic for relief of pain.
   a. In internal organs by reflex action.
   b. In muscles and joints by counterirritation.
2. *Derivation* to increase blood flow peripherally in order to relieve congestion internally.
3. *Stimulation*
   a. To increase blood flow to part; a short (3 to 5 min.), intense application which may be followed by cold.
   b. To stimulate certain functions of internal organs and to decrease others.

(28)

    c. To promote leukocytosis.

    d. To promote diaphoresis.

    e. To produce tissue warming and relaxation in preparation for massage, exercise, electrical stimulation, or ultrasound.

4. *Sedative* (mild heat 6 to 10 min.)

    a. To relieve nervous states such as insomnia and nervous tension.

    b. To relieve spasm (mild to moderate heat) by increasing circulation and by release of nervous tension.

Equipment

1. Fomentation tank heated by boiling water or steam.
2. Three complete fomentations (3 wet packs and 3 dry covers).
3. Basin of ice water.
4. Two Turkish towels.

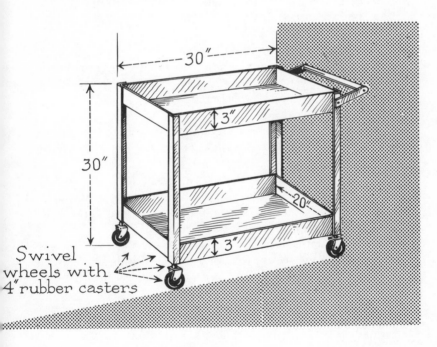

5. One or two compress cloths, usually washcloths or bath mittens.
6. Bath blanket or sheet.
7. Patient's hospital gown.

Procedure

1. *Important considerations*
   a. *Remember* that the duration and frequency in changing fomentations depend upon the desired effect to be obtained.
   b. Be especially careful with thin or aged persons, and children. *Avoid chilling.*
   c. Take care *not* to burn unconscious, paralyzed, diabetic, edematous patients, or patients with impaired local circulation.
   d. Do not apply fomentations where there is danger of hemorrhage or suspected malignancy.
   e. Be careful not to spread infection.
2. *Preparation*
   a. Explain procedure to the patient.
   b. Have the room warm and free from drafts. Secure privacy.
   c. Have the patient remove clothing and drape with a sheet. For the bed patient (room treatment), cover with bath blanket and remove hospital gown.
   d. Be sure patient's feet are warm. If heat is not ordered (arteriosclerosis, diabetes, etc.) cover the feet with a warm blanket.
   e. For treatment of postoperative areas, cover all dressings with a plastic protector before applying the fomentation.
   f. A plastic cover may also be used to help retain heat if the application is ordered for long periods.
   g. If cerebral congestion may occur, have cold compresses to apply to the neck as well as to the head. In heart disease or with pulse 80 or above, place an ice bag over heart.
3. *Treatment*
   a. Have all equipment ready.
   b. Cover with a bath towel the part to be treated.

    c. Apply fomentation to the area as indicated. To relieve congestion have the fomentation extend over a large area. For local effect make the fomentation the area size.

    d. Use intensity of heat as indicated by the patient's condition and effect to be obtained.

    e. Protect sensitive parts and bony prominences.

    f. Lift the fomentation and rub the hand firmly over the towel to absorb moisture if unbearably hot.

    g. Apply a cold compress to the head and/or neck; change every 2 to 4 minutes. Use an ice bag to heart if needed.

    h. Give three fomentations unless otherwise indicated, drying the part well before each additional application. Change the towel if necessary.

    i. After the last fomentation rub the area with a cold compress and dry thoroughly.

    j. In case of severe pain have the fomentation as HOT as can be tolerated. Omit cold in extreme pain such as pleurisy, renal colic, dysmenorrhea.

    k. Warm alcohol may be used for astringent effect and to cool patient.

4. *Completion of treatment*

    a. Leave patient comfortable and free from perspiration.

    b. Remove equipment and leave area tidy.

    c. Make a record of the treatment, frequency, and length of application.

    d. Report the effect of the treatment, the reaction of the patient, and any deviation of results noted.

References

1. Abbott, G. K.; Moor, F. B.; and Nelson, K. J.: *Physical Therapy in Nursing Care*. Washington, D.C., Review and Herald Pub. Assn., 1941, pp. 74-81.
2. Bierman, W.; and Licht, S.: *Physical Medicine in General Practice*. New York, Paul B. Hoeber, 1947, pp. 49-50.
3. Finnerty, G. B.; and Corbitt, T.: *Hydrotherapy*. New York, Frederick Ungar Pub. Co., 1960, pp. 103-107.

4. Fuerst, E. V.; and Wolff, L. V.: *Fundamentals of Nursing.* Philadelphia, Lippincott, 1946, p. 364.
5. Harmer, B.; and Henderson, V.: *Textbook of the Principles and Practice of Nursing.* New York, Macmillan, Fifth Edition, 1957, pp. 633, 640-645.
6. Krusen, F. H.; Wakim, K. G.; Leden, U.; Martin, G. W.; and Elkins, E. C.: "Effect of Hot Packs on Peripheral Circulation." *Archives of Physical Medicine* 31:145 (March), 1950.

CHEMICAL PACK (Hydrocollator) (Chem. Pk.)

Definition

Moist heat applied by means of a preheated chemical pack of silica gel.

Effects and indications

1. To relieve pain.
2. To increase blood flow to an area.
3. To relax muscle spasm.

Equipment

1. Chemical pack.
2. Electrical heating unit or basin of boiling water and heat source.
3. One or two bath towels.
4. Plywood square for carrying pack (15 x 15 inches).
5. Plastic covering.
6. (Method 1) Two fomentation covers.
7. (Method 2) One large beach towel (approximately 36 x 68 inches).

Procedure

1. *Important considerations*
   a. The electric heating units should be plugged in at least one hour before use.

b. Water level in heating unit should be maintained by adding water each day as necessary.

c. The dry pack must be soaked for one hour, then heated
fifteen minutes.

d. Packs should never be allowed to dry after they have been
moistened, since they harden and are difficult to soften
again.

e. There should be 6 or 7 thicknesses of towel or cover
between the patient's skin and the moist pack.

f. Do not allow patient to lie upon the pack.

2. *Preparation for treatment*

a. The pack should be placed in the tank with one set of
loops uppermost for easy removal. The pack will be more
effectively heated if placed vertically (sections up and
down) in the heating unit.

b. Method I

(1) Spread one fomentation cloth on the work area for
cover.

(2) Place a second fomentation cloth folded in fourths in
the center of the cover. This will make *five* thicknesses of wrap under the pack when placed over a
folded towel.

(3) Remove the pack from the tank and place on the
folded fomentation cloth. Wrap with the outer fomentation cover.

(4) The plywood square can be used to carry the pack to
the patient.

c. Method II

(1) Fold the beach towel across into 5 layers. Fold lower
edge about one fifth of length. Then bring upper
edge of towel to first fold. Fold again to make 5 thicknesses.

(2) Place the pack on center of the folded towel. Cover
with plastic to retain heat. The ends of the folded
towel can be brought over the pack.

(3) The folded towel can be used for one, two, or even

three packs for application to the spine or an extremity.

(4) The pack is placed over a folded towel to make *seven* thicknesses between the pack and the patient.

3. *Treatment*
   a. The patient's clothing should be removed.
   b. Drape and make comfortable.
   c. Fold the Turkish towel in half, place over the area to be treated.
   d. Place the pack on the area over the folded towel so that *seven* thicknesses are between the pack and the patient.
   e. Heat lasts about 30 minutes. The pack may be covered with a folded towel or plastic.
   f. Sponge the area with a cold compress or apply alcohol and dry thoroughly.

4. *Completion of treatment*
   a. Give follow-up care as ordered.
   b. See that the patient is free from perspiration.

References

1. Brown, A. F.: *Medical Nursing.* Philadelphia, W. B. Saunders Co., 1959, p. 695.
2. Finnerty, G. B.; and Corbitt, T.: *Hydrotherapy.* New York, Frederick Ungar Pub. Co., 1960, pp. 123-125.
3. Harmer, B.; and Henderson, V.: *Textbook of the Principles and Practice of Nursing.* New York, Macmillan, 1955, p. 639.

THE PARAFFIN BATH (Par. B.)

Definition

The local application of melted paraffin to the skin surface.

Effects

1. Hyperemia and other effects of local heat.
2. Preparation of the skin for massage by making it smooth, soft, and pliable.

Indications

1. Arthritic joints, stiff joints after fractures or sprains.
2. Bursitis, fibrositis, and tenosynovitis after the acute phase is past.

Equipment

1. Commercial paraffin bath or double boiler for home use (see note).
2. Commercial paraffin (1 pint of mineral oil to 5 pounds of paraffin for home use).
3. Taylor dairy thermometer capable of registering up to 150° F. (A cork top will keep the thermometer floating.)
4. Plastic for wrapping.
5. Basin for used paraffin.

Procedure

1. *Important considerations*
   a. Examine the skin for open lesions and unhealed scars and skin infections. Never use the paraffin bath when there is an open lesion.
   b. Use great care in treating old, weak, debilitated individuals. (Use a rack in the tank—do not allow patient to touch the bottom of the tank.)
   c. Paraffin bath should not be used in the treatment of peripheral vascular diseases.

2. *Preparation*
   a. Wash the part before treatment.
   b. Instruct the patient to hold the fingers or toes in relaxed position without moving in order to avoid cracks in the paraffin "glove."
   c. Have the patient remove the clothing and drape to avoid damp clothing due to perspiration.
   d. Seat the patient comfortably.

3. *Treatment*
    a. Temperature 122° to 130° F. or with a film formed over the top of the paraffin.
    b. Dip body part 6 to 12 times, allowing for cooling after each dip.
    c. After dipping, either leave part in paraffin 15 to 20 minutes or wrap part in plastic and cover with towel to preserve heat 15 to 20 minutes.
    d. If both hands are to be treated, dip one hand first, and remove and wrap in plastic while the other hand is done. The effect is prolonged by contralateral heating.
    e. Remove the paraffin (glove) and place in a basin. The "glove" may be used for finger exercise (squeezing and kneading) or cleaned and replaced in the tank.
4. *Completion of treatment*
    a. Give follow-up care as prescribed.
    b. Chart the treatment and reaction.
    c. Care of paraffin and tank:
        (1) Add water in the basin in which peeled paraffin glove is placed, heat to the boiling point to remove perspiration. Remove from the fire, let cool. When cold, and paraffin is hardened, remove from basin and dry and replace in the paraffin tank.
        (2) Keep the lid and framework of tank free from paraffin.
        (3) When not in use, keep tank covered at all times.
        (4) To sterilize paraffin in the tank, heat to a temperature of 180° to 200° F.

Note: For home use a double boiler made by Vollrath Company, Sheboygan, Wisconsin, is obtainable. It is shown in the Hotel Section of the Hospital Equipment Catalog; wholesale price, $5.90; size, base 7¾ quart, insert 7 quart.

References

1. Abbott, G. K.; Moor, F. B.; and Nelson, K. J.: *Physical Therapy in Nursing Care.* Washington, D.C., Review and Herald Pub. Assn., 1941, pp. 459, 460.

2. Finnerty, G. B.; and Corbitt, T.: *Hydrotherapy.* New York, Frederick Ungar Pub. Co., 1960, pp. 118-123.
3. Margolin, H.: "A Method of Keeping the Paraffin Bath Free of Sediment." *The Phys. Ther. Rev.* 41:271 (April), 1961.
4. Stimson, C. W.; Rose, G. B.; and Nelson, P. A.: "Paraffin Bath as Thermotherapy: An Evaluation." *Arch. Phys. Med. and Rehab.* 39:219 (April), 1958.

HOT FOOT BATH (H. Ft. B. or Hft. B.)

Definition

A local immersion bath covering the feet and ankles at temperatures ranging from 100° to 115° F.

Effects and indications

1. Local and reflex increase in blood flow through the feet and entire skin surface producing decongestion in internal organs and brain (derivative effect).
   a. To relieve congestive headache.
   b. To relieve chest congestion.
   c. To relieve pelvic congestion.
   d. To stop epistaxis.
2. General warming of body
   a. To prepare the patient for general application of heat.
   b. To prepare the patient for tonic procedures.
   c. To produce sweating, when prolonged.
   d. To help prevent or abort a common cold.
3. To aid relaxation and comfort.
4. Treatment of local inflammation of feet.

Equipment

1. Foot tub or container large enough and deep enough; 5-gallon can or dishpan may be used.
2. Thermometer if available; if not, test water temperature with elbow, temperature 103° to 115° F.
3. Sheet or bath blanket.

4. Turkish towel, cold compress if needed.
5. Material for protection of the bed—rubber sheet or plastic.
6. Pitcher or dipper to add hot water.

Procedure

1. *Important considerations*
   a. Use care in adding hot water to avoid burning.
   b. Hot foot bath should not be used in peripheral vascular disease unless specifically ordered by physician.
   c. Not recommended for frostbite.
2. *Preparation*
   a. Explain procedure to the patient.
   b. Have room warm and free from draft.
   c. Assemble materials.
   d. Protect bedding.
   e. The patient may lie or sit, properly draped.
3. *Treatment*
   a. Have the water 103° F., deep enough to cover ankles.
   b. Assist the patient to place his feet in the tub. Place your hand in water to reassure the patient.
   c. Drape patient and cover tub.
   d. Add hot water from time to time to increase the temperature to tolerance; never exceed 115° F.
   e. Continue for 10 to 30 minutes; check the reaction for perspiration.
   f. Use cold compress to the head as indicated. Renew often.
   g. When finished, pour cold water over the feet. Remove from the tub and dry thoroughly.
   h. If the patient is perspiring, give an alcohol rub or other cooling measure and dry thoroughly.
4. *Completion of treatment*
   a. Give follow-up care as prescribed.
   b. Be sure patient is warm and comfortable.
   c. Remove equipment.
   d. Record treatment, temperature, time, also reaction.

References

1. Abbott, G. K.; Moor, F. B.; and Nelson, K. J.: *Physical Therapy in Nursing Care.* Washington, D.C., Review and Herald Pub. Assn., 1941, p. 113.
2. Bierman, W; and Licht, S.: *Physical Medicine in General Practice.* New York, Hoeber, 3d ed., 1957, p. 36.
3. Harmer, B.; and Henderson, V.: *Textbook of the Principles and Practice of Nursing.* New York, Macmillan, 1955, p. 639.
4. Finnerty, G. B.; and Corbitt, T.: *Hydrotherapy.* New York, Frederick Ungar Pub. Co., 1960, pp. 10, 48.

WHIRLPOOL BATH (Wpl. B.)

Definition

A partial immersion bath in which the water is agitated and mixed with air to be directed against the affected area.

Effects

1. Cleanses and stimulates wound healing.
2. Sedative—relieves pain and relaxes spasm.
3. Conductive heat and gentle massage are combined to stimulate circulation.
4. Softens tissues preparatory for massage, stretching, and exercise.

Indications

1. Amputation stumps.
2. Sprains and contusions after the first thirty-six hours.
3. Postoperative orthopedic conditions.
4. Peripheral vascular disease: venous (including indolent ulcers) not over 105° F.; arterial not over 93° F.
5. Peripheral nerve injuries.
6. Arthritis and fibrositis.
7. Burns.

Equipment

1. Whirlpool tank (approximately forty gallons).
2. Tub for contrast application if needed.
3. Stool or bench.
4. Material for a cold compress (turban and/or cravat).
5. Ice bag if needed.
6. Drape sheet or gown.
7. Halter (or gown) and trunks if patient is to be immersed.
8. Bath thermometer.

Procedure

1. *Important considerations*
   a. Remove all dressings if possible before starting the agitator. (If dressings need to be loosened, hold with forceps until they can be removed.) See that no dressings are left in the tank, as they will clog and damage the agitator.
   b. Caution—avoid overheating the patient who has peripheral vascular disease or peripheral nerve injury.
   c. If the treated area is sensitive, agitation of the water should be reduced until better tolerated.
2. *Preparation*
   a. Fill the whirlpool bath to desired depth at the desired temperature, 105° to 110° F., or 93° F.
   b. The whirlpool should be adequately grounded, either with a 3-way plug or separate ground wire to a water pipe or radiator.
   c. Add a tablespoonful of hexachlorophene G-11 or other antiseptic to the water.
   d. For infected wounds add 10 grams of sodium sulfathiazole per 8 gallons.
   e. For burns use normal saline (isotonic) solution. To a 40-gallon tank add 3 pounds of salt. (1 gal. = 8 lbs. 40 x 8 x .9% = 320 x .9% = 2.88 lbs. salt.)
   f. If the arm is to be treated place a chair by the tub. If treating a leg or foot, seat the patient on elevated chair or bench, or on a treatment table with back supported.

3. *Treatment*
   a. Apply a cold compress (cravat to neck and/or turban to head).
   b. Inspect the part before immersion. Adjust height of agitator and force of circulating water.
   c. Treatment time 10 to 25 minutes. May be alternated with cold immersion for a contrast application.
   d. Treatment may be concluded with a pour of cool or cold water over the part (vasomotor response).
4. *Completion of treatment*
   a. Dry as necessary for further treatment.
   b. Chart the time, the temperature, the reaction, and progress.
   c. Thoroughly wash and rinse the tank.

References

1. Abbott, G. K.; Moor, F. B.; and Nelson, K. J.: *Physical Therapy in Nursing Care.* Washington, D.C., Review and Herald Pub. Assn., 1941, pp. 116-117.
2. Bierman, W.; and Licht, G.: *Physical Medicine in General Practice.* New York, Hoeber, 1957, pp. 39, 40.
3. Brown, A. F.: *Medical Nursing.* Philadelphia, W. B. Saunders Co., 1957, p. 697.
4. Finnerty, G. B.; and Corbitt, T.: *Hydrotherapy.* New York, Frederick Ungar Pub. Co., 1960, pp. 61-71.
5. Kovacs, R.: *Manual of Physical Therapy.* Philadelphia, Lea and Febiger, 1951, pp. 211, 212.
6. Licht, S.: *Therapeutic Heat.* New Haven, Elizabeth Licht, 1958, p. 345.

THE SITZ BATH (Z. B.)

Definition

The sitz bath is a partial bath covering the pelvic region, given in a specially constructed tub.

Effects and indications

1. Hot Sitz (105° to 115° F. for 2 to 10 minutes).
   a. Analgesic and stimulant to the pelvic circulation.

    b. Indicated in dysmenorrhea, acute and chronic cystitis, chronic pelvic inflammatory disease, prostatitis, and after cystoscopy and hemorrhoidectomy.

2. Cold Sitz (55° to 75° F. for 2 to 10 minutes with friction).

    a. Increases the tone of smooth muscle of the uterus, bladder, and colon. Lessens tendency to bleeding from the uterus and the lower bowel and rectum.

    b. Indicated in subinvolution of the uterus, metrorrhagia, atonic constipation, and for general tonic effect.

3. Contrast Sitz.

    a. Hot phase: 105° to 115° F., 3 minutes.
       Cold phase: 55°to 85° F., 30 seconds.
       Three changes.

    b. Increase the pelvic circulation and tone of smooth muscle of the pelvic organs.

    c. Indicated in chronic pelvic inflammatory disease, chronic prostatitis, atonic constipation, fistula in ano, following rectal surgery.

4. The hot half bath may be substituted for the hot sitz bath in home treatment for upper respiratory infections, congestive types of headaches, chronic pelvic inflammatory disease, prostatitis, dysmenorrhea, and acute and chronic cystitis.

Equipment

1. Materials for H. Ft. B.
2. Materials for C. Comp. Hd. (turban) and C. Comp. Nk.
3. Sitz tub.
4. Bath thermometer.
5. Bath towels.
6. Hospital gown.
7. Rubber ring if needed.
8. Shower cap.
9. Stool for foot tub if needed.
10. Ice bag if needed.

Procedure

1. *Important considerations*
   a. Prolonged heat changes effects obtained (see note).
   b. Check the patient's pulse.
   c. Check the water temperature.
2. *Preparation for treatment*
   a. Explain the procedure to the patient.
   b. Have the patient void.
   c. Prepare the tub (rubber ring for patients following rectal surgery).
   d. Prepare a hot foot bath 105° F. (increase as indicated).
3. *Treatment*
   a. Assist the patient, as necessary, into tub. Place the feet in the foot bath.
   b. Drape so that the patient is not exposed.
   c. Apply cold to the head and neck; watch for fainting. Ice bag over the heart may be necessary.
   d. Increase and maintain the temperature as ordered. When adding hot water, place the hand between the stream and the patient to prevent burning.
   e. Conclude the hot sitz by cooling the bath to neutral three minutes or by pail pour to the hips.
   f. Assist the patient out of the tub and with drying.
   g. The patient may have a cleansing spray bath following the sitz.
4. *Completion of treatment*
   a. Assist the patient as needed (dressing, wheelchair, etc.).
   b. Have the patient rest.
   c. Record the treatment and the effects.

Note: "The cutaneous branches of the external iliac are widely dilated, diverting blood from the internal viscera. The hot foot bath, by dilating the branches of the external iliac, still further drains the portal circulation. At temperatures above 110° F., especially if the bath is continued beyond 3 or 4 minutes, the effect is to excite the pelvic circulation, and to concentrate the blood in this portion of the body."—Kellogg: *Rational Hydrotherapy,* 1928, page 769.

References

1. Abbott, G. K.; Moor, F. B.; and Nelson, K. J.: *Physical Therapy in Nursing Care.* Washington, D.C., Review and Herald Pub. Assn., 1941, pp. 117-120.
2. Finnerty, G. B.; and Corbitt, T.: *Hydrotherapy.* New York, Frederick Ungar Pub. Co., 1960, pp. 51-57.
3. Fuerst, E. V.; and Wolff, L. V.: *Fundamentals in Nursing.* Philadelphia, Lippincott, 1959, p. 412.
4. Harmer, B.; and Henderson, V.: *Textbook of the Principles and Practice of Nursing.* New York, Macmillan, 1957, 5th ed., p. 639.

COLD COMPRESS (C. Comp.)

Definition

A cloth wrung from cold or ice water which may be applied to any part of the body surface.

Effects and indications

1. Vasoconstriction—the blood flow is decreased locally and distally.
2. Relief of pain due to edema or trauma.
3. Prevent and relieve congestion.
4. Antipyretic when applied over a large area (at least one fourth of body surface).
5. Applied over the heart, slows rate, increases the force, and raises the arterial blood pressure.

Equipment

1. Compress may be a washcloth or a hand towel, the size depending on the part to be treated.
2. Basin for cold or ice water.
3. Plastic or rubber sheeting for bed, pillow, or where needed.

SITZ-BATH TECHNIQUES

Sitz	Temperature	Time	Finish	Effect	Therapeutic Indications
Hot (a)	105° to 115° F. Hft. B.—110° to 117° F. (2° hotter than Z.)	3 to 10 min.	Cool Z. to neutral 3 min. (cooling may be omitted).	Analgesic.	Dysmenorrhea, acute or chronic cystitis, after cystoscopy or hemorrhoidectomy, sciatica, urinary retention, prostatitis, fibrositis.
Hot (b)	105° to 115° F. Hft. B.—110° to 117° F.	3 to 10 min.	Pail pour to hips 65° to 55° F.	Acceleration of blood flow.	Chronic pelvic inflammatory disease, low back pain.
Cold (with friction)	55° to 75° F. Hft. B.—105° F.	2 to 8 min. (2 to 4 min.)	Friction to hips promotes reaction.	Stimulation of circulation and muscle tone.	Subinvolution of uterus, atonic constipation.
Contrast (alternate hot and cold)	H. 105° to 115° F. C. 55° to 85° F. Hft. B.—105° to 115° F.	H.—2 min. C.—30 sec. (3 complete changes)	Finish with cold.	Powerful acceleration of blood flow.	Chronic pelvic inflammatory disease, atonic constipation, low back pain, prostatic hypertrophy.
Hot ½ bath (home procedure)	100° to 110° F.	3 to 10 min.	1. Cool to neutral. 2. Pail pour 65° to 55° F.	Analgesic, acceleration of blood flow, derivative.	Sinusitis, upper respiratory infection, headache.

(45)

Procedure

1. *Important considerations*
   a. The reflex effect of a cold compress should always be kept in mind.
   b. Some patients cannot tolerate moist cold over the sinuses.
   c. The cold compress is often applied as a turban to the head or a cravat to the neck with general heating procedures.
2. *Preparation*
   a. See that the patient is in a comfortable position.
   b. Do not cover a cold compress.
3. *Treatment*
   a. Apply and press firmly.
   b. Avoid chilling the patient.
   c. Renew frequently, every 1 to 5 minutes.
   d. Dry thoroughly.
4. *Completion of treatment*
   a. Hair, pillows, and bedding should be dry to avoid chilling.

References

1. Abbott, G. K.; Moor, F. B.; and Nelson, K. J.: *Physical Therapy in Nursing Care.* Washington, D.C., Review and Herald Pub. Assn., 1941, pp. 87-91, 62.
2. Harmer, B.; and Henderson, V.: *Textbook of the Principles and Practice of Nursing.* New York, Macmillan, 1957, pp. 649, 650.
3. Finnerty, G. B.; and Corbitt, T.: *Hydrotherapy.* New York, Frederick Ungar Pub. Co., 1960, pp. 108, 109.

THE HEATING COMPRESS (Heat. Comp.)

Definition

The heating compress is a mild prolonged application of moist heat of several hours' duration.

Effects and indications

1. To relax muscles.
2. To relieve pain of sore throat or rheumatic joints.
3. To relieve abdominal distress (moist abdominal bandage).

Equipment

1. One or two thicknesses of loosely woven cotton cloth wide enough to cover the area and long enough for one circumference of the part.
2. Outer covering of one thickness of part-wool flannel long enough and wide enough to completely cover cotton cloth and extend ½ inch on each side.

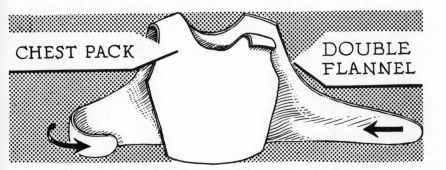

CHEST PACK   DOUBLE FLANNEL

3. Safety pins to secure the compress in place.
4. Basin of water at temperature desired (usually tap water).

Procedure

1. *Important considerations*
   a. If medication is to be used, apply it first.
   b. Wring cotton cloth so that it does not drip when applied.
   c. Apply compress smoothly and quickly to avoid chilling.
   d. Wrap snugly to exclude air and pin securely.
   e. Take care that compress is not so tight as to interfere with circulation, respiration, or joint movement.
   f. Do not cover with plastic. This interferes with the hyperemic reaction.
   g. The patient's ability to react to cold applications is an important factor.

2. *Preparation for treatment*
   a. Tell the patient the application is cold but warms up by body reaction after the dry cover is in place.
   b. Patient should be thoroughly warm before the compress is applied; give hot foot bath if necessary.
3. *Treatment*
   a. Apply compress snugly with flannel. Pin securely.
   b. Leave in place several hours or overnight.
4. *Completion of treatment*
   a. Remove the compress, rub the area quickly with a cold washcloth.
   b. Dry thoroughly and see that the patient is warm and comfortable.
   c. Chart the treatment, time applied, and reaction.

Heating compress to throat

1. Used in pharyngitis, laryngitis, tonsillitis.
2. May be applied dry with camphorated oil.
3. In children use head band to hold compress snugly at ears.

Heating compress for joints

1. To relieve joint pain and inflammation in rheumatic fever, chronic arthritis, or synovitis.
2. If reaction is poor the compress may be applied dry or with medication to area.

Heating chest pack

1. For a mild derivative effect in chronic bronchitis, whooping cough, or pneumonia.
2. The choice of a dry or moist pack will depend on the vitality of the patient and the desired result.
3. A fitted chest pack may be made with pieces for front and back as for a vest, so that it may be fastened snugly over the shoulders and under the arm.

4. It may be desirable to apply the moist cloth to a portion of the chest only (the upper bronchial area) with the fitted dry chest pack.

Moist abdominal bandage

1. Used in insomnia, central nervous exhaustion, constipation, nausea of pregnancy, and other gastrointestinal disturbances.
2. The compress should be 8 or 9 inches wide and long enough to reach 1½ times around the abdomen.
3. The dry flannel should be twelve inches wide.
4. The lower edge of the bandage should be below the iliac crests.
5. The dry flannel should be fitted to the patient by pinning darts on each side.
6. When applied at night it is usually dry by morning.

References

1. Abbott, G. K.; Moor, F. B.; and Nelson, K. J.: *Physical Therapy in Nursing Care.* Washington, D.C., Review and Herald Pub. Assn., 1941, pp. 91-99, 349, 377, 380, 438.
2. Bierman, W.; and Licht, S.: *Physical Medicine in General Practice.* New York, Hoeber, 1957, pp. 48, 49.
3. Finnerty, G. B.; and Corbitt, T.: *Hydrotherapy.* New York, Frederick Ungar Pub. Co., 1960, pp. 107-110.

THE ICE PACK (Ice Pk.)

Definition

A local application of cold over a covered body segment.

Effects

1. Relief of pain.
2. Prevention of ecchymosis and swelling.
3. Decrease of blood flow, local metabolism, and inflammation.

Indications

1. Early treatment of sprains, contusions, soft tissue injuries.
2. Acute bursitis.
3. Acute joint inflammation of rheumatic fever, rheumatoid arthritis, and acute infectious arthritis.
4. Immediate treatment of burns.

Equipment

1. White heavy wool flannel (preferably stitched around the edge). Use a piece at least 12 x 12 inches for the shoulder or knee and 8 x 8 inches for the elbow or ankle.
2. One or two Turkish towels.
3. Safety pins.
4. Plastic—one or two pieces.
5. Finely crushed ice, or snow.

Procedure

1. *Important considerations*
   a. Observe reaction of the skin to avoid tissue injury.
   b. Apply the pack specified time—usually 30 minutes at intervals of 2 to 4 hours as prescribed.
2. *Preparation*
   a. Explain the purpose of cold application for condition treated.
   b. Spread the Turkish towel out on a flat surface; over the towel spread finely crushed ice to make a layer one inch thick; fold towel and pin together securely. Make the pack large enough to cover the area to be treated.
3. *Treatment*
   a. Apply the pack over the flannel-covered area, then cover with plastic and a Turkish towel or bandage to hold in place.
   b. Use another piece of plastic or a piece of rubber sheeting to protect bedding.

 c. Continue the application 30 minutes.
 d. Remove the pack, dry the area carefully, and observe reaction.
 e. Cover or bandage area to avoid chilling the patient.
4. *Completion of treatment*
 a. Chart treatment, duration, and reaction.
 b. Be sure the patient is comfortable and not chilled.

References

1. Abbott, G. K.; Moor, F. B.; and Nelson, K. J.: *Physical Therapy in Nursing Care.* Washington, D.C., Review and Herald Pub. Assn., 1941, pp. 88, 457, 467.
2. Finnerty, G. B.; and Corbitt, T.: *Hydrotherapy.* New York, Frederick Ungar Pub. Co., 1960, p. 129.

CONTRAST LOCAL APPLICATIONS

Definition

The application of alternate heat and cold to a local area.

Effects and indications

1. As an analgesic through acceleration of local circulation.
2. To stimulate healing in local injuries with ecchymosis (contusions).
3. To relieve muscle stiffness and pain due to trauma or strain.
4. To stimulate healing in wound infections.

Equipment

1. Fomentations for application of heat (Turkish towels wrung from hot water may be used).
2. Two Turkish towels to be wrung from ice water (smaller towels may be used for smaller areas).
3. Plastic to cover dressings in wound infections.
4. Patient's gown.

Procedure

1. *Important considerations*
   a. Alternate applications produce both circulatory and thermic reactions.
   b. Maximum effects are obtained with short, intense, alternate applications of about equal length.
   c. In cases of wound infection cover the area with a piece of plastic to avoid moisture on dressings.

2. *Preparation for treatment*
   a. Have three fomentations prepared or available as needed.
   b. Assemble all materials.
   c. Assist the patient into a comfortable position and drape the area. Avoid getting the bed linen wet.

3. *Treatment*
   a. Cover area to be treated with a Turkish towel (use a piece of plastic under the towel over dressings).
   b. Apply the fomentation as hot as can be tolerated for 3 minutes.
   c. Wring a Turkish towel from ice water and apply directly to the area (1 minute) after removing the fomentation and towel. Have second Turkish towel wrung out of ice water. Change 3 times.
   d. Next, apply a fomentation for 3 minutes.
   e. Make 3 complete applications of contrast—heat 3 minutes and cold 3 minutes—for a total of 18 minutes.

4. *Completion of treatment*
   a. Note condition of the treated area. Give follow-up care as indicated.
   b. In wound infections the dressings may need to be changed.
   c. Assist the patient as needed.

References

1. Abbott, G. K.; Moor, F. B.; and Nelson, K. J.: *Physical Therapy in Nursing Care.* Washington, D.C., Review and Herald Pub. Assn., 1941, p. 346.

2. Kellogg, J. H.: *Rational Hydrotherapy.* Philadelphia, Davis, 1928, pp. 640, 816-821, 842.
3. Krusen, F. H.: *Physical Medicine.* Philadelphia, W. B. Saunders Co., 1941, p. 510.
4. Moor, F. B.: "Hydrotherapy for Local Injuries and Infections." *Archives of Physical Therapy,* Nov., 1941, p. 645.

CONTRAST BATHS (Cont. B.) (H. & C. Lg. B.— H. & C. Arm B.)

Definition

The immersion of a body part alternately in hot and cold water.

Effects

1. Alternate contraction and dilatation of blood vessels (vascular exercise).
2. Marked increase of blood flow locally and reflexly. Derivative effect.
3. Increased local metabolism. Hastens healing.

Indications

1. Impaired venous circulation, indolent ulcers.
2. Infections (2 to 3 times a day), lymphangitis.
3. Sprains, strains, and trauma (after 48 hours).
4. Fractures and other orthopedic conditions.
5. Rheumatoid arthritis.
6. Indurative edema.
7. Congestive headaches by derivation with immersion of the feet and legs.

Equipment

1. Two containers large enough to allow the part to be submerged.
2. Thermometer.
3. Drape sheet or gown.

5—M.H.M.

4. Turkish towels.
5. Cold compress (ice bag if needed).
6. Disinfectant if needed.

Procedure

1. *Important considerations*
   a. Contraindicated in malignancies or where there is a tendency to hemorrhage.
   b. If a large part of the body is treated, use a cold compress to the neck and head (ice bag to the heart if the pulse is 80 or above).
   c. Do not have the temperature of the hot water above 110° F. Extremes of heat and cold should not be used in peripheral vascular disease.
   d. Begin hot immersion at lower limits, increasing the temperature during application. With subsequent treatments gradually reach the maximum temperature limits.
   e. A disinfectant should be used in water for an open wound. (See Appendix, page 160.)
2. *Preparation for treatment*
   a. Assemble materials. Have room warm and free from drafts.
   b. Explain procedure. Check pulse.
   c. Assist the patient as necessary. Remove bandages, dressings, etc. Examine the area.
3. *Treatment*
   a. Place the part to be treated in hot water 103° to 110° F. for 3 to 4 minutes.
   b. Place in cold water (tap or ice water) for ½ to 1 minute.
   c. While in cold water, increase temperature of hot water to at least maintain beginning temperature.
   d. Check pulse every 5 minutes, apply cold compress (cravat) to neck, and ice bag to heart if needed.
   e. Make 6 to 8 changes (20 to 30 minutes) and end in cold. (Rheumatoid arthritis end with hot water.)
   f. Dry thoroughly.
   g. Give cooling measure if indicated.

4. *Completion of treatment*
   a. Give follow-up care as ordered.
   b. Chart treatment, temperature, time, and reaction.
   c. Adequate cleaning of equipment is essential. (See Appendix, pages 159, 160.)

References

1. Abbott, G. K.; Moor, F. B.; and Nelson, K. J.: *Physical Therapy in Nursing Care.* Washington, D.C., Review and Herald Pub. Assn., 1941, pp. 114-116.
2. Bierman, W.; and Licht, S.: *Physical Medicine in General Practice.* New York, Hoeber, 3d ed., 1957, pp. 36-38.
3. Finnerty, G. B.; and Corbitt, T.: *Hydrotherapy.* New York, Frederick Ungar Pub. Co., 1960, pp. 9, 57, 58.

ALTERNATE HOT AND COLD TO HEAD (H. & C. Hd.)

Definition

The use of heat and cold to improve cerebral circulation by vascular stimulation—heat is applied to the lower extremities to provide added derivation.

Effects and Indications

To relieve certain selected headaches such as headaches due to the passive congestion of the common cold, nervous and muscular tension, and certain headaches due to trauma.

Equipment

1. A covered oblong ice pack filled with finely chopped ice; two ice bags may be used.
2. Two compresses; Turkish towels may be used.
3. Two sets of fomentations (for a room treatment 6 fomentations will be required to make 3 changes).
4. Material for hot foot bath.
5. Turkish towels.

6. Basin of ice water.
7. Shower cap.
8. Drape sheet or bath blanket.
9. Hospital gown.

Procedure

1. *Important considerations*
   a. Explain the procedure to the patient.
   b. Have the patient in supine position.
   c. Alternate heat and cold to the head should not be used in headache due to hypertension and only in carefully selected cases of trauma.
2. *Preparation for treatment*
   a. Protect the bed with a rubber sheet.
   b. A pillow may be used.
   c. Have the ice pack long, narrow, and not too bulky to fit the neck adequately.
3. *Treatment*
   a. Hot foot bath 105° to 115° F. Begin 105°F. Increase as needed.
   b. Place a fomentation covered with a Turkish towel under the cervical spine and to sides of the neck; two hot water bags may be used.
   c. Place a compress wrung from ice water on the face, covering the top of the head and ears. Press down firmly over the forehead and the temporal arteries; *renew every minute* 3 times.
   d. Replace the fomentation to the neck with long, narrow ice pack or with two covered ice bags (one to each side of neck).
   e. Replace the cold compress to the face with a fomentation or Turkish towel wrung from hot water; cover the ears and forehead but do not cover the nose, allowing the patient to breathe cool air. Protect the eyes from excessive heat and do not press down on the fomentation.

f. Continue the alternations for 3 complete sets of heat and cold.

g. Holding the feet above a foot tub, pour cold water over feet and dry thoroughly.

h. Cool face by sponging with a cold compress.

i. Dry thoroughly, especially the hair.

4. *Completion of treatment*

a. Have the patient rest at least 30 minutes after treatment. Avoid chilling.

b. Record treatment and reaction.

Note: The value of this treatment is evident only when heat is also applied to the feet to secure a derivative effect.

Skeleton outline of procedure

1. Fo. Nk.	cc. face	3 min.
Ice Nk.	fo. face	3 min.
2. Fo. Nk.	cc. face	3 min.
Ice Nk.	fo. face	3 min.
3. Fo. Nk.	cc. face	3 min.
Ice Nk.	fo. face	3 min.

Total time   18 minutes

References

1. Abbott, G. K.; Moor, F. B.; and Nelson, K. J.: *Physical Therapy in Nursing Care.* Washington, D.C., Review and Herald Pub. Assn., 1941, p. 84.
2. Kellogg, J. H.: *Rational Hydrotherapy.* Philadelphia, Davis, 1928, pp. 840-844.

HOT AND COLD TO CHEST (H. & C. Ch.)

Definition

The use of alternate applications of heat and cold to the chest to relieve congestion by vascular stimulation. If heat is applied to the lower extremities systemic derivation will also be achieved.

Effects and indications

1. To prevent chest congestion following anesthesia in some surgical cases.
2. To stimulate respiration and recovery from anesthesia.
3. To prevent circulatory stasis following anesthesia.
4. To aid in the relief of congestion due to a chest cold.

Equipment

1. Five Turkish towels.
2. Two compress cloths.
3. Two small rubber sheets.
4. Bath blanket.
5. Patient's bath basin with a large piece of ice.
6. Five fomentations in container well wrapped to minimize heat loss.

Procedure

1. *Important considerations*
   a. Patients who have had major surgical procedures may be given this treatment in the evening of day of surgery, morning and evening of the first postoperative day, and morning of the second postoperative day—under routine or standing orders.
   b. Exceptions usually listed include eye surgery, tonsillectomy, thyroidectomy, mastectomy and chest surgery, and all genitourinary surgery.
   c. Contraindicated for children under 12 years, unconscious persons, areas of impaired sensation or circulation, paralyzed areas.
   d. Use special care in treating older patients and diabetics.
2. *Preparation for treatment*
   a. Explain procedure to the patient.
   b. Assemble materials.

c. If the treatment is given in the patient's room protect the bedside table.

d. Protect bed and drape patient with a bath blanket.

3. *Treatment*

a. Assist the patient to turn on his side.

b. Place a rubber sheet, one fomentation and bath towel lengthwise as close as possible beside the patient's back.

c. Have the patient turn back on the fomentation. Rub the hand under the shoulders and hips to make certain the fomentation is smooth and not too hot.

d. Cover the chest with a towel; over this place a fomentation. Be careful that the fomentation is not too hot over sensitive areas. Cover patient with a bath blanket.

e. Place a rubber sheet, a fomentation, and a Turkish towel under the patient's feet. Wrap well. Cover with a bath blanket.

f. Remove the fomentation from chest. Have the patient take a deep breath while the chest is rubbed briskly with ice, covering the area about two times.

g. Dry area thoroughly and apply the next fomentation.

h. Make 3 applications of heat and cold to the chest, finishing with cold.

i. Remove the fomentations from the feet and back and cool the parts with alcohol. Dry thoroughly.

j. The entire treatment should be given briskly, in 10 to 15 minutes.

4. *Completion of treatment*

a. Leave the patient comfortable and free from perspiration.

b. Remove the equipment and leave the area tidy.

c. Make a record of the treatment and condition after treatment.

Reference

Kellogg, J. H.: *Rational Hydrotherapy*. Philadelphia, Davis, 1928, pp. 840-847.

ROUTINE HOT AND COLD TO THE CHEST (H. & C. Ch.)

Routine

1. Given to all major surgical patients four times.
   a. Evening of day of surgery.
   b. Morning of first postoperative day.
   c. Evening of first postoperative day.
   d. Morning of second postoperative day.
   Except in the following, unless specifically ordered:
   a. Tonsillectomy.
   b. Thyroidectomy.
   c. Mastectomy.
   d. All genitourinary surgery, such as prostatectomy, nephrectomy, etc.
   e. Chest surgery.
   f. Cataract and other eye surgery.
2. For vein ligation, dilatation, and curettage and other minor procedure given on the night following surgery only.
3. Given to orthopedic patients by surgeon's order.

Effects

1. Marked increase in blood flow locally and reflexly.
2. Stimulation of respiration.

Equipment

1. Paper towels to protect bedside table.
2. Five Turkish towels.
3. Washcloth for compress.
4. Two small rubber sheets.
5. Bath blanket.
6. Patient's bath basin with a large piece of ice.
7. Five fomentations.

Procedure

1. Explain the treatment.

2. Screen the patient.
3. Clear the bedside stand.
4. Drape the patient with a bath blanket.
    a. In morning treatments remove the top linen and place on a chair.
    b. In afternoon treatments fan fold the top linen to foot of bed.
5. Check to see if the patient has towels, rubber sheets, and washcloth at bedside.
6. Take the patient's washbasin to the ultility room and get ice chips and a large smooth piece of ice. If it is rough, it may be smoothed by rubbing it on fomentation tank. Add a little water.
7. Secure any necessary linen.
8. Obtain 3 fomentations, wrapping and rolling them in the proper manner.
    a. Protect your arm with an extra wrapper when removing fomentations from the tank.
    b. Place a fomentation on the center of the wrapper and fold edges over quickly.
    c. Roll tightly with the singly wrapped side inside.
9. Take the equipment to bedside.
10. Have the patient turn on side.
11. Place the rubber sheet, fomentation, and towel lengthwise beside the patient's back.
12. Push the edges of all three as close to the patient as possible.
13. Have the patient turn on his back, making certain that he is centered on the fomentation. Rub your hand under the shoulders and hips to make certain the fomentation isn't too hot.
14. Place a towel over chest.
15. Place a fomentation over the area, with the singly wrapped part next to the towel. Rub your hand under the fomentation and lift it if it is too hot.
16. Cover with a bath blanket.
17. Place a rubber sheet, fomentation, and towel on the foot of

the bed. Place the patient's feet on the towel. Wrap the
edges around the feet. Cover with a bath blanket.

18. Check in same manner to be sure fomentation on the feet
    is not too hot. If any of the fomentations are too hot or too
    damp, use an extra towel.
19. Wring a washcloth from ice water and place on the forehead.
20. Leave fomentation on chest 3 minutes.
21. Get a second one ready before removing the first.
22. Warn the patient that cold will be applied. Remove fomen-
    tation, ask the patient to take a deep breath, and rub ice
    briskly over his chest, covering the area about 2 times.
23. Dry the area thoroughly.
24. Give 3 applications of heat and cold to the chest, finishing
    with cold.
25. Remove the fomentations from the feet and back and return
    them to the fomentation tank.
26. Straighten the bed and unit and replace all equipment. Hang
    the rubber sheet and the towels on a rod at head of the bed.
27. Chart.
    a. Chart:
       (1) Time.
       (2) Treatment.
       (3) Reaction, particularly if unusual.
       (4) Signature.

Precautions

1. The entire treatment should be completed in 10 to 15 minutes
   —given briskly. Do not try to do anything else at the same
   time! Stay with the patient except when getting the fomentations. Do not talk too much—let him relax.
2. Check frequently by placing your hand next to skin to be sure
   the fomentation isn't too hot.
3. If fomentation is still unduly hot or damp, use an extra Turkish towel.
4. Use special care in treating aged patients, diabetics, etc.

TECHNIQUE OF FRICTIONS, SPRAYS, AND DOUCHES

COLD MITTEN FRICTION (C. M. F. or Cmf.)

Definition

An application of cold water with friction of Turkish towel, friction mitts, or luffa mitts.

Effects

1. Stimulates circulation and metabolism.
2. Increases white blood cell activity and antibody production.
3. Stimulates neuromuscular tone.
4. Vasomotor tonic.

Indications

1. Convalescence after fevers.
2. Hyperthyroidism, preoperative, and postoperative.[1]
3. Central nervous exhaustion, paralysis agitans.
4. Hypochromic anemia.
5. To build up resistance as part of a graduated hydrotherapy program.

Equipment

1. Two sheets or two bath blankets.
2. Two mitts.

3. Pail or large basin of cold water, temperature 40° to 70° F.
4. Bath towels.
5. Material for hot foot bath and cold compress for the head.

Procedure

1. *Important considerations*
   a. Make sure the patient is warm, especially his feet.
   b. Do not expose more than one part of body at one time; avoid chilling.
   c. Avoid skin lesions.
   d. The patient must be warm and dry after treatment.
   e. Success of the cold mitten friction depends on the speed and vigor of treatment.
   f. "Best of all means for training to react to cold."[2]
2. *Preparation*
   a. Protect the bed from dampness; use a bath blanket under the patient if necessary.
   b. Explain the treatment and purpose.
   c. Assemble materials.
   d. Water temp. 60° to 70° F.; lower the temp. 1° to 2° each treatment to 40° to 50° F.
3. *Treatment*
   a. Do one part at a time, extremities first, chest, then back.
   b. Wring mitts quickly from cold water and rub part vigorously 5 to 8 seconds.
   c. Quickly cover part with towel and dry with friction.
   d. Cover the area and proceed with next body segment.
   e. Tonic or stimulating effects depend on
      (1) The temperature of water.
      (2) Repeated dipping of mitts 1 to 4 times.
      (3) The duration of application.
      (4) The vigor of friction applied.
4. *Completion of treatment*
   a. Be sure the patient is warm and dry.
   b. Make a record of the treatment and the patient's reaction.

References

1. Abbott, G. K.; Moor, F. B.; and Nelson, K. G.: *Physical Therapy in Nursing Care.* Washington, D.C., Review and Herald Pub. Assn., 1941, pp. 101-104, 320, 399.
2. Kellogg, J. H.: *Rational Hydrotherapy.* Philadelphia, Davis, 1928, pp. 308, 642-647.

SALT GLOW (S. G. or Sgl.)

Definition

The application of wet salt with rubbing to the patient's skin.

Effects and indications

1. Tonic and stimulating.
2. It produces vigorous stimulation of the peripheral circulation.
3. It builds up resistance as a stimulant for persons who do not react well to cold. It takes less body reactivity to produce a reaction than does the cold mitten friction.

Equipment

1. Basin containing 1 to 2 lbs. salt.
2. Foot bath—104° F.
3. Stool (if patient sits).
4. Turkish towels and washcloth.
5. Drape sheet or gown.
6. Shower cap and thongs.

Procedure

1. *Important considerations*
   a. Salt glow should not be given if there is skin disease present.
   b. Pressure of the movement should be even, taking care over bony prominences and sensitive areas. Heavier friction may be used over buttocks.

    c. Rapid movements may be more irritating to the skin than stimulating to the circulation.

2. *Preparation*
    a. Avoid drafts.
    b. Moisten salt so that it sticks together.
    c. Explain purpose of the treatment.
    d. Drape patient as needed during the procedure.

3. *Treatment*
    a. Have all equipment ready.
    b. Wet patient's skin with water; take both hands full of moistened salt; apply to an extremity and give friction to tolerance.
    c. Start with the extremities—then do the chest, the back, and the buttocks; the abdomen may be omitted.
    d. If seated, have the patient stand to do the buttocks.
    e. Remove the salt by spray or pail pour; wash off *all* salt.
    f. Dry the patient thoroughly.

4. *Completion of treatment*
    a. Observe the skin reaction.
    b. Give follow-up care as ordered.
    c. Report results such as the skin reaction.

References

1. Abbott, G. K.; Moor, F. B.; and Nelson, K. J.: *Physical Therapy in Nursing Care.* Washington, D.C., Review and Herald Pub. Assn., 1941, p. 108.
2. Finnerty, G. B.; and Corbitt, T.: *Hydrotherapy.* New York, Frederick Ungar Pub. Co., 1960, pp. 88-91.

COMPLETE ALCOHOL RUB (Alc. R.)

Definition

    The application of rubbing alcohol to the surface of the body.

Effects and indications

1. For a cooling effect after general or local applications of heat.
2. To lower body temperature in fevers.

3. To protect pressure areas by the astringent effect on the skin.
4. To refresh the patient when a bath is not given.

Equipment

1. Rubbing alcohol or 95% pure grain alcohol diluted to make a 70% solution (or alcohol ⅔–water ⅓).
2. Basin of hot water to warm the bottle of alcohol if necessary.
3. Bath blanket.
4. Turkish towels to protect the bedding.

Procedure

1. *Important considerations*
   a. Pour alcohol into the cupped hands to avoid chilling the patient.
   b. Be sure such areas as the neck, axilla, under the breast, umbilicus, groin, and gluteal cleft are dry.
2. *Preparation for treatment*
   a. Assemble equipment.
   b. Replace top bedding with a bath blanket and drape the patient.

Treatment

1. Rub upper extremities first.
   a. Apply the alcohol with an upward stroke, returning with rotary movements to cover the entire surface. Repeat as needed.
   b. For cooling effects use short alternating strokes to aid evaporation of the alcohol (avoid pawing movements).
   c. Finish with three superficial strokes from the shoulder to the hand, using both hands to cover the surface. (Be sure that patient is dry.)
2. Rub chest.
   a. Apply alcohol with one long stroke up to the shoulders, returning with rotary movements to the lateral part of chest. Repeat as needed.

b. Use short, brisk strokes (for evaporation of alcohol) beginning at the shoulder, first one side and then the other side.

c. Finish with superficial strokes downward from the shoulders on both sides.

3. Rub lower extremities.

a. Modify the movements as used for upper extremity, being sure to cover the posterior surface of the leg and thigh thoroughly.

4. Rub back.

a. Assist the patient to turn on the side or abdomen, placing a pillow under the patient's lower chest and abdomen.

b. Apply alcohol with both hands from the buttocks to the shoulders—follow with firm rotary movement to the shoulders, scapulae, ribs, hips, and buttocks. Repeat as needed.

c. Apply circular kneading with right hand over coccygeal area.

d. Finish with superficial stroking from the shoulders to the buttocks using both hands to cover the surface. Stroke the spine from the neck to the buttocks with hands alternating.

Completion of treatment

1. Leave the patient comfortable and in good alignment.
2. In treatment of pressure areas record the present skin condition.
3. Take the temperature at stated intervals to check on fever reduction. Chart.

References

1. Abbott, G. K.; Moor, F. B.; and Nelson, K. J.: *Physical Therapy in Nursing Care.* Washington, D.C., Review and Herald Pub. Assn., 1941, p. 109.
2. Finnerty, G. B.; and Corbitt, T.: *Hydrotherapy.* New York, Frederick Ungar Pub. Co., 1960, p. 36.
3. Fuerst, E. V.; and Wolff, L. V.: *Fundamentals of Nursing.* Philadelphia, Lippincott, 1956, p. 181.
4. Harmer, B.; and Henderson, V.: *Textbook of the Principles and Practice of Nursing.* New York, Macmillan, 1955, pp. 335, 336.

SPRAY (Spr.)

Definition

The spray is an application of water from multiple needle spray heads striking the entire body surface, except the head and feet, horizontally from four directions.

Effects and indications

1. Cleansing for ambulatory and neurological patients.
2. As a tonic procedure with or without a previous application of heat.

Equipment

1. One or two sheets.
2. Two or three Turkish towels.
3. Shower cap for women.
4. Thong sandals for ambulatory patients.
5. Stool.
6. Metal chair on casters if needed for neurological patients.

Procedure

1. *Important considerations*
   a. Be aware of the patient's problems in doing self-care; encourage and assist as needed.
   b. Avoid danger of falling; ambulatory patients may wear thong sandals.
2. *Preparation for treatment*
   a. Have the patient properly draped, either ambulatory or in a special chair.
   b. Turn on the spray and regulate the temperature to the patient's comfort, 94° to 100° F.
3. *Treatment*
   a. Have the patient step into or wheel into the spray.
   b. With a washcloth, soap and rinse the body well (if the

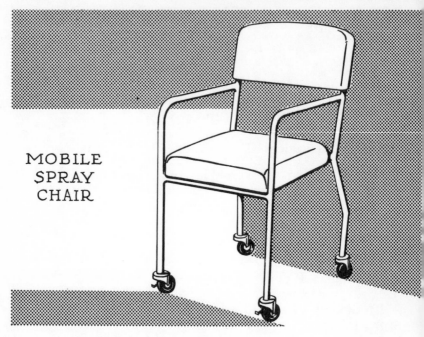

MOBILE
SPRAY
CHAIR

patient is able, encourage him to bathe himself); assist as needed for complete care.

    c. Check and maintain the water temperature about 98° F.

    d. Turn off the spray, and assist the patient as necessary for drying; be sure the feet are well dried.

    e. Fan the patient with a sheet if desirable and indicated.

4. *Completion of treatment*

    a. Give follow-up care as prescribed.

    b. Be sure the patient is warm and comfortable.

References

1. Abbott, G. K.; Moor, F. B.; and Nelson, K. J.: *Physical Therapy in Nursing Care.* Washington, D.C., Review and Herald Pub. Assn., 1941, pp. 150-159.
2. Bierman, W.; and Licht, S.: *Physical Medicine in General Practice.* New York, Hoeber, 1957, pp. 41, 42, 51-55.
3. Brown, A. F.: *Medical Nursing.* Philadelphia, W. B. Saunders Co., 1957, p. 630.

4. Fuerst, E. V.; and Wolff, L. V.: *Fundamentals of Nursing*. Philadelphia, Lippincott, 1959, p. 233.
5. Harmer, B.; and Henderson, V.: *Textbook of the Principles and Practice
   of Nursing*. New York, Macmillan, 5th ed., p. 331.
6. Krusen, F. H.: *Physical Medicine*. Philadelphia, W. B. Saunders Co.,
   1941, pp. 482-484.
7. Finnerty, G. B.; and Corbitt, T.: *Hydrotherapy*. New York, Frederick
   Ungar Pub. Co., 1960, pp. 79-88.

SPRAY (Spr.)

The effect of the spray may be varied by regulation of the
temperature and duration.

Neutral spray (Neut. spr.)

1. *Effect:* Sedative, relaxing.
2. *Temperature:* Begin 100° to 102° F., drop steadily to 97°
   to 94° F.
3. *Time:* 3 to 5 minutes after reaching neutral temperature.
4. *Completion:* Dry with a minimum of friction and no fanning.

Hot spray (H. spr.)

1. *Effect:* Cleansing, preparation for cold spray or douche.
2. *Temperature:* Begin 100° F., gradually raise the temperature
   to tolerance (110° to 115° F.), hold 1 to 2 minutes, cool
   rapidly (90° to 85° F.).
3. *Time:* 1 to 2 minutes after reaching the patient's tolerance of
   heat.
4. *Completion:* Friction with a towel, fan with a sheet.

Graduated spray (Grad. spr.)

1. *Effect:* Cooling, not tonic or stimulating.
2. *Temperature:* Begin at 100° F., quickly raise the temperature
   to tolerance (110° to 115° F.), maintain 1 to 3 minutes,
   gradually lower to 100° F., maintain 1 to 3 minutes, then
   lower to 90° F. (or 94° F.) and maintain 1 to 3 minutes.
3. *Time:* 7 to 9 minutes.
4. *Completion:* Dry with some friction.

5. *Important considerations*
   a. The patient should be in a state of heat conservation; he should not feel cold at any time.
   b. There is great danger of chilling; extreme care should be taken to avoid chilling during and after the spray.

Hot and cold spray (H. & C. spr.)

1. *Effect:* Vigorous tonic.
2. *Temperature:* In the hot and cold spray there are three changes as follows:
   a. Begin at 100° F. and quickly increase temperature to 110° F. for 1 minute; then quickly lower to 90° for ½ to 1 minute.
   b. Increase hot phase to 112° F. for 1 minute; decrease cold phase to 85° F. for ½ to 1 minute.
   c. Increase hot phase to 115° F. for 1 minute; end spray with neutral 94° F. for 2 to 3 minutes.
3. *Time:* 4 to 6 minutes.
4. *Completion:* Dry with friction.
5. *Important considerations*
   a. The hot and cold spray is a progressive program in vascular exercise.
   b. It has a definite fatigue-relieving effect.

Allergy spray (Blomquist)

1. *Effect:* This procedure was originated by Dr. Olov Blomquist for the treatment of vasomotor rhinitis, hay fever, and asthma. Its exact mode of action has not been determined. It is known that the vasomotor reactions of the nasal mucosa are abnormal in vasomotor rhinitis and hay fever and that they are improved by the alternate hot and cold spray. This may at least partially explain the favorable response to the hot and cold spray. Another possible mode of action is an increase in steroid production through stimulation of the pituitary-adreno cortical mechanism.

SPRAY ➤	MINUTES (°F ➤)	TIME ➤	DRYING ➤	EFFECT ➤
NEUTRAL		Begin 100°–102°F Drop steadily to 97°–94°F Hold 3–5 minutes	Dry without friction or fanning	Sedative Relaxing
HOT		Gradually raise temp. to tolerance Hold 2 minutes Cool rapidly to 90–85°F	Friction with towel Fan with sheet	Cleansing Preparation for cold spray or douche
GRADUATED		Quickly raise temp. to tolerance 110°–115° Maintain 1–3 min. Gradually lower to 100° & maintain for 3 min. Then lower to 94°F Should not feel cool	Dry with some friction Patient should be in state of heat conservation. Danger of chilling	Cooling, not tonic or stimulating Should not feel cold at any time
HOT and COLD		Begin 100°F Hot phase 1 minute Cold " ½ to 1 " Three changes End neutral	Dry with friction Vascular exercise	Vigorous tonic

2. *Temperature*
   a. Begin at 100° F., increase rapidly to 108° to 110° for 3 minutes, then decrease rapidly to 85° for 2 minutes.
   b. Change rapidly to 112° to 114° F. for 3 minutes, then rapidly to 75° for 2 minutes.
   c. Change rapidly to 116° to 118° F. for 3 minutes, then rapidly to 65° for 2 minutes.
3. *Time:* About 15 minutes.
4. *Completion:* Dry with friction.
5. *Important considerations*
   a. The patient should have a 20-minute rest period after the spray.
   b. The patient should get a vigorous reaction to the allergy spray. If the reaction is not satisfactory, the spray may have to be modified.

PERCUSSION DOUCHE (Perc. D.) (Scotch Douche)

Definition

A column of water directed against some portion of the body.

Effects

Effects vary according to the area treated, and the mass, pressure, temperature, and duration of the column of water striking the body.

Equipment

Same as for sprays, with the addition of percussion hose and controls.

Procedure

1. *Important considerations*
   a. Ideally the spray should be on while the douche is given. However, physical layout of spray and douche area may make this impossible.

b. Effects vary according to the area treated, the mass, pressure, temperature, and duration.

c. The cerebral circulation is better regulated and better results are obtained if all applications begin and end with the feet.

d. A definite pattern should be learned and followed.

e. The operator's finger should be kept in contact with water as it comes from the nozzle.

f. With a steady hand, apply douche accurately to part to be treated; the column of water should be kept moving.

g. Watch the thermometers constantly.

h. The breasts should be protected by covering with one arm. The free arm may be used to hold the grab bar.

i. The percussion douche should not be used in:

   (1) Cardiac and renal disease.

   (2) Arteriosclerosis.

   (3) Exophthalmic goiter.

   (4) Hypertension.

   (5) Nervous irritability.

   (6) Neuritis.

   (7) Varicose veins—avoid pressure on involved areas.

   (8) Severe illness.

j. The stream should be fanned over the popliteal area when treating back, and fanned over the front of the body. The exception is the front of the thighs, where jet may be used.

2. *Preparation*

   a. Explain the procedure to the patient.

   b. Turn on the spray and regulate the temperature to the patient's comfort (94° to 100° F.).

3. *Treatment*

   a. Beginning at the feet, apply the douche as indicated in accompanying drawing, fanning at areas indicated.

   b. Complete douche as ordered; turn off.

   c. Turn off the spray. Assist the patient as needed for drying (dry feet well).

   d. Fan the patient with a sheet if desirable and indicated.

4. *Completion of treatment*
   a. Give follow-up care as prescribed.
   b. Be sure the patient is warm and comfortable.

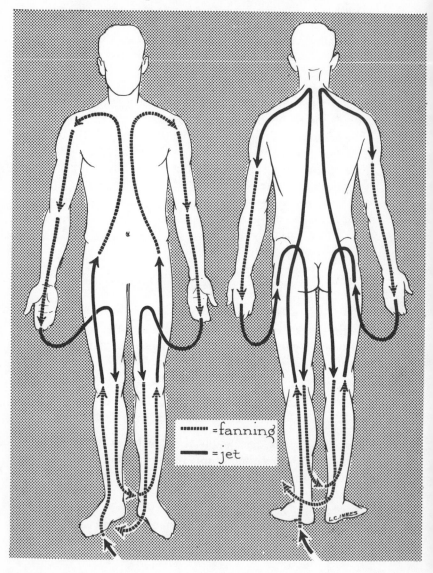

Hot percussion douche (H. douche)

1. *Effects*
   a. Derivation due to dilatation of the cutaneous vessels (large areas).
   b. Reflex dilatation of deep vessels (small area).
   c. Stimulation.
   d. Without percussion (fan jet with finger) relief of pain and irritation, neuralgia, sciatica.
2. *Temperature:* 105° to 118° F.
3. *Time:* Hot 2 to 5 minutes, followed by very brief cold (5 to 15 seconds) 60° to 90° F.

Neutral douche (Neut. douche)

1. *Effects*
   a. Sedative (the jet should be fanned with the finger).
2. *Temperature:* 94° to 97° F.
3. *Time:* 3 to 6 minutes.

Contrast douche (H. & C. douche)

1. *Effects*
   a. Vigorous circulatory stimulant.
   b. Powerful tonic and stimulant to neuromuscular system.
2. *Temperature*
   a. Heat, 110° to 115° F.
   b. Cold, 90° to 85° F. (See spray chart, page 73.)
3. *Time*
   a. Heat, 1 minute.
   b. Cold, ½ to 1 minute. Usually 3 changes.

References

1. Abbott, G. K.; Moor, F. B.; and Nelson, K. J.: *Physical Therapy in Nursing Care.* Washington, D.C., Review and Herald Pub. Assn., 1941, p. 154.
2. Finnerty, G. B.; and Corbitt, T.: *Hydrotherapy.* New York, Frederick Ungar Pub. Co., pp. 85, 86.
3. Krusen, F. H.: *Physical Medicine.* Philadelphia, W. B. Saunders Co., 1941, pp. 482, 483.

TECHNIQUE OF GENERAL THERMAL PROCEDURES

CLEANSING TUB BATH (Tub B.)

Definition

A bath given for cleansing purposes.

Effects and indications

1. "Cleanliness is the first step in the prevention of both mental and physical disease."
2. Circulatory tonic, relieves fatigue.
3. It refreshes the patient in mind and body and relieves discomfort from position, heat, moisture, and other causes.
4. Given to cleanse from external dirt, such as dust, infectious material, metabolic waste excreted by the skin and decomposing substances which are irritating and give rise to disagreeable odors.

Equipment

1. Two Turkish towels.
2. Washcloth.
3. Soap or detergent.
4. Patient's gown and slippers.
5. Air pillow or folded bath towel.

(78)

Procedure

1. *Important considerations*
   a. A cleansing tub bath should be given only if the patient's condition permits.
   b. The room should be warm and free from drafts.
   c. Always remain with the patient as a safety measure.
   d. Grab bars are always necessary so that the patient can help himself in and out of the tub.
   e. If the skin is to be thoroughly cleansed, use a detergent such as hexachlorophene (G-11).
2. *Preparation*
   a. Prepare the bath water 100° to 105° F.
   b. Have all materials ready.
3. *Treatment*
   a. Assist the patient into the tub.
   b. Place a Turkish towel over the patient.
   c. Using washcloth and soap, assist the patient to wash every part of the body.
4. *Completion of treatment*
   a. Assist the patient out of tub.
   b. Dry thoroughly.
   c. Give follow-up treatment as ordered.

References

1. Harmer, B.; and Henderson, V.: *Textbook of the Principles and Practice of Nursing*. New York, Macmillan, 1939, pp. 281, 285, 288.
2. Shafer, K. N.; Sawyer, J. R.; McCluskey, A. M.; and Lifgren, E. E.: *Medical and Surgical Nursing*. Saint Louis, C. V. Mosby Co., 1958, p. 146.

BATHTUB TRANSFERS

1. One attendant: Place the patient on a stool the same height as the tub, near the end of the tub. Swing the patient's feet over into the tub. Have the patient hold the grab bar or the opposite side of the tub. Stabilize the patient by holding

under the arms to assist sitting down in the tub. Reverse the procedure for getting out of the tub.

2. When more assistance is needed in getting out of the tub, two attendants may be needed. Drain the tub and partially dry the patient. Place a dry towel under the hips for a lifter. While one attendant lifts the patient at the hips a second attendant (standing behind the patient) lifts by holding under the arms. With coordinated efforts the patient is lifted to the edge of the tub and transferred to the stool. Then the legs are swung out of the tub by one attendant while the patient is supported by the second attendant.

3. Teaching a patient to move from a wheelchair into a tub and back to the chair: "The seat of the chair is covered with a waterproof square and a large Turkish towel. The patient, dressed in a bathrobe, is directed to bring the chair as close as possible to the tub, facing it. After braking the chair, he lifts each foot into the tub, pushing up on the arms of the chair. He moves toward the tub so that the buttocks are partly on the edge of the chair and partly on the rim of the tub. Leaning forward and grasping the tub on each side or a bar on the side, the buttocks can be lowered into the water. A paralyzed leg can be lifted and flexed so that the foot and the lower part can be bathed. Bracing the foot against one end of the tub or resting against the back steadies the body.

"To get out, the process is reversed. With the body braced against the back of the tub, it is brought out of the water by pushing up on the rim. The buttocks rest first on the edge of the tub and with another push are moved over on the seat of the chair. After unlocking the brakes, the chair is moved out six inches and the legs are removed singly from the tub. The body is dried and the gown replaced."

Reference

Harmer, B.; and Henderson, V.: *Textbook of the Principles and Practice of Nursing.* New York, Macmillan, 5th ed., 1955, p. 492.

FULL IMMERSION BATH

Baths	Temperature	Time	Procedure	Finish	Effects and Indications
Hot tub bath	100° to 106° F. begin at 98° F.	2 to 20 minutes	1. Cold water to drink. 2. C. comp. to head and neck. 3. Ice bag to heart.	1. Cool bath. 2. Cold pour. 3. Graduated spray.	1. Cleansing. 2. Relief of spasm. 3. Pyrexia, short. 4. Sweating, prolonged. 5. Rheumatoid arthritis home treatment.
Neutral	94° to 97° F.	15 to 20 minutes	1. Temp. variation. a. Season of year. b. Patient's skin temperature. 2. Add warm water after 10 minutes to maintain temperature.	1. Cool bath. 2. No friction with drying.	1. Sedative and relaxing. 2. Preparation for rest or to precede other treatment.
Continuous flow	98° F.	1 or more hours	1. Hammock and restraint may be necessary. 2. Remove the patient for skin care and bowel hygiene.	Skin care.	1. Mania and other disturbed psychiatric states.

NEUTRAL TUB BATH (Neut. B.)

Definition

Immersion of the body in a tub of water at a neutral temperature (94° to 98° F.).

Effects and indications

1. Sedative in central nervous exhaustion, insomnia, nervous irritability. The sedative effect is due to the fact that the neutral temperature is not stimulating and the water prevents external skin stimuli.

Equipment

1. Bathtub (5½ or 6 ft.) and bath thermometer.
2. Basin of ice water, compress cloths.
3. Two Turkish towels and a bath mat if desired.
4. Two sheets and shower cap.
5. Air pillow or a folded Turkish towel for the patient's head.

Procedure

1. *Important considerations*
   a. The temperature will vary with the condition of the patient, especially with regard to the skin temperature, season of the year, temperature of the room, etc.
   b. All heat treatments should precede the neutral bath.
   c. If the patient is to be in the bath longer than 4 hours, lubricate the skin with a lanolin cream before the bath.
2. *Preparation*
   a. Fill the tub with neutral water to cover the patient (94° to 98° F.).
   b. Have all materials ready.
   c. The room should be quiet, with subdued light.
   d. The bath should feel comfortably warm; hence the patient's sensation is a better guide than a thermometer.

3. *Treatment*
   a. Assist the patient into the tub, placing an air pillow or folded Turkish towel under the head. Have the patient comfortable without strain.
   b. Cover with a Turkish towel, or cover the tub with a sheet.
   c. Instruct the patient to lie quietly and relax; use a cold compress as needed.
   d. If the bath lasts longer than 15 to 20 minutes, add more warm water to maintain the temperature.
   e. Stay with the patient. Do not talk unless by so doing you can keep patient quiet.
   f. Duration: From 15 to 20 minutes, to 3 or 4 hours.
   g. Cool bath 2 or 3 degrees if necessary.
   h. Assist the patient out of the tub.
   i. Dry quickly without friction or unnecessary rubbing.
   j. Assist the patient with dressing as needed.
4. *Completion of treatment*
   a. The patient should have an undisturbed rest period of at least 30 minutes.

References

1. Abbott, G. K.; Moor, F. B.; and Nelson, K. J.: *Physical Therapy in Nursing Care.* Washington, D.C., Review and Herald Pub. Assn., 1941, p. 121.
2. Finnerty, G. B.; and Corbitt, T.: *Hydrotherapy.* New York, Frederick Ungar Pub. Co., 1960, pp. 40, 41, 45.
3. Krusen, F. H.: *Physical Medicine.* Philadelphia, W. B. Saunders Co., 1941, pp. 476-488.
4. Harmer, B.; and Henderson, V.: *Textbook of the Principles and Practice of Nursing.* New York, Macmillan, 1957, pp. 620, 621.

HUBBARD TANK (Hub. Tank)

Definition

A specially constructed full-immersion tub with turbine for administering underwater exercises with neutral or mild heat application or mild fever therapy.

Effects

1. The bath is relaxing and cleansing.
2. Buoyancy of the water is an aid to exercise.
3. Mild heating facilitates stretching.
4. Turbine increases circulatory effects and aids mobilization.
5. Saline and brine solutions aid in treatment of burns and decubitus ulcers.

Indications

1. Rheumatoid arthritis.
2. Neuromuscular conditions such as hemiplegia, poliomyelitis, Parkinson's disease, multiple sclerosis, and cerebral palsy.
3. Postoperative orthopedic conditions.
4. Burns and decubitus ulcers.

Equipment

1. Hubbard tank.
2. Turbine or agitator.
3. Stretcher canvas and backrest.
4. Mechanical lift or hoist.
5. Cart (stretcher or gurney).
6. Bath thermometer.
7. Linen.
8. Halter, loincloth, and/or trunks.
9. Swim cap if needed.
10. Cold compresses.

Procedure

1. *Important considerations*
   a. The buoyancy of the water aids the patient in exercise.
   b. Hydrostatic pressure of the water benefits circulation.
   c. The turbine may be added for hydromassage effect.
   d. The patient should not be left alone.
   e. Avoid cross infections; adequate cleaning of tank is important.

f. Patients with communicable disease, skin rash, or common cold should have tank therapy postponed.

g. In acute conditions, kidney diseases, cardiac problems, anemias, tuberculosis, Hubbard tank therapy may be contraindicated.

h. Temperature, duration, and exercise program vary with the condition treated and the tolerance of the patient.

2. *Preparation for treatment*
   a. Have the tank ready.
   b. Explain the procedure to the patient to minimize apprehension; the first treatment may well be an orientation.
   c. Prepare the patient with halter, loincloth, or trunks, and/or hospital gown.

3. *Procedure for use in poliomyelitis* (early convalescent period)
   a. Bath temperature 98° F.
   b. Place the patient in the tank.
   c. Have patient perform the prescribed exercises for about 10 minutes.
   d. Raise temp. to 102° F. (100° F. for children under 12).
   e. The patient rests 7 to 8 minutes; the turbine may be applied to indicated areas.
   f. Lower temperature to 98° F.
   g. Stretching by the therapist, 10 minutes.
   h. Remove the patient from the tank; dry thoroughly.
   i. Transfer to a treatment table for dressing.

4. *Procedure for fractures, hemiplegias, etc.*
   a. Bath temperature 90° to 98° F., depending on condition of the patient; higher temperatures for relief of pain and stretching contractures; lower temperatures for active motion exercise programs. Temperatures: for flaccid paralysis, 90° F.; spastic, 100° F.
   b. Prepare the patient and assist into the tank.
   c. The turbine, if available, may be directed to specific areas.
   d. After a warming period or application of the turbine, stretching procedures, range-of-motion exercises, passive and/or active, are carried out.

e. Time: 20 to 30 minutes.

f. Remove the patient from the tank, dry thoroughly, and transfer to a treatment table for other procedures and/or dressing or transfer to a dry stretcher for return to his room.

g. Be very cautious with the hoists and lift in the transfer of patients, to avoid injury. If necessary use a three-man lift to transfer the patient from the wet stretcher to the treatment table.

h. Have the patient rest after the treatment.

i. Keep record of the patient's progress, range of motion, muscle strength, relief of pain, etc.

References

1. Abbott, G. K.; Moor, F. B.; and Nelson, K. J.: *Physical Therapy in Nursing Care.* Washington, D.C., Review and Herald Pub. Assn., 1941, p. 460.
2. Bierman, W.; and Licht, S.: *Physical Medicine in General Practice.* New York, Hoeber, 1957, pp. 30, 31.
3. Finnerty, G. B.; and Corbitt, T.: *Hydrotherapy.* New York, Frederick Ungar Pub. Co., 1960, pp. 71-79.
4. Kovacs, R.: *Manual of Physical Therapy.* Philadelphia, Lea and Febiger, 1951, pp. 212-214.
5. Licht, S.: *Therapeutic Heat.* New Haven, Elizabeth Licht, vol. 2, pp. 188, 189, 220, 221, 377, 378.
6. Licht, S.: *Therapeutic Exercises.* New Haven, Elizabeth Licht, vol. 3, ch. 10, pp. 280-289.

HUBBARD TANK FOR RHEUMATOID ARTHRITIS (Hub. Tank)

Effects and indications

1. To induce a mild fever.
2. Effects of heat to joints and adjacent muscles.
3. Medium for range-of-motion exercises to prevent deformities.

Equipment

1. Hubbard tank.
2. Stretcher canvas and backrest.

3. Mechanical lift or hoist.
4. Cart (stretcher or gurney).
5. Bath thermometer.
6. Linen.
7. Halter and loincloth or trunks.
8. Swim cap if needed.
9. Cold compress or turban for head.
10. Ice bag if needed.

Procedure

1. *Important considerations*
   a. Watch the patient closely; temperature may rise quickly (see note).
   b. Use a cold compress (turban) to the head to prevent overheating and headache.
   c. May give fluids after the temperature rises.
   d. Do not leave the patient unattended; two attendants are needed.
   e. Treatment is usually given 2 or 3 times per week.
2. *Preparation*
   a. Explain purposes of treatment to minimize apprehension and obtain full cooperation of the patient.
   b. Determine and record the patient's temperature, pulse, and respiratory rates.
   c. Prepare the patient with a halter and loincloth or trunks.
3. *Treatment*
   a. Place the patient in the Hubbard tank with the water temperature at 98° to 100° F.
   b. After 3 to 5 minutes increase the tank temperature gradually to 104° to 106° F. and maintain at that level as indicated below.
      (1) First treatment: Maintain the tank temperature at 104° to 106° F. until the patient's temperature rises 1° F.
      (2) 2d trt.: Maintain the tank temperature at 104° to 106° F. until the patient's temperature rises 2° F.

(3) 3d and subsequent trt.: Maintain the tank temperature at 104° to 106° F. until patient's temperature reaches 101° to 102° F. .

c. When the indicated temperature has been reached, lower the tank temperature to the beginning level.

d. Put all joints through maximum range of motion to the point of pain.

e. Remove from the tank to the treatment table, cover, allow to cool to almost normal body temperature. Finish treatment by massage (mostly kneading and stroking) to the muscles of the extremities, with friction as tolerated around the joints.

f. On removal from tank, the patient may be wrapped in blankets to prolong effect of mild fever if prescribed.

g. Check pulse rate while patient is in the tank and use an ice bag to heart if indicated.

h. Keep a record of successive progressive treatments.

Note: "General heating puts severe demands on pulmonary ventilation." "General applications of heat are more debilitating than local heat."—Licht, et al, Therapeutic Heat, vol. 2, pp. 377, 378.

References

1. Kovacs, R.: Manual of Physical Therapy. Philadelphia, Lea and Febiger, 1951, pp. 212-214.
2. Krusen, F. H.: Physical Medicine. Philadelphia, W. B. Saunders Co., 1941, p. 476.

HUBBARD TANK FOR MULTIPLE SCLEROSIS AND PARKINSON'S DISEASE (Hub. Tank)

Effects and indications

1. Lessen muscle spasm.
2. Relaxation of clonus.
3. Improve coordination.
4. Lower body temperature—mild hypothermia.

Equipment

1. Hubbard tank with agitator.
2. Linen as needed.
3. Halter and loincloth and/or shorts.

Procedure

1. *Important considerations*
   a. Suggested temperature range of bath, 70° to 80° F. Suggested time, 10 minutes, increased to 20 minutes as tolerated.
   b. Temperature of bath may need to be graduated to tolerance. First treatment begin at 96° to 98° F., lower to 80° F. if tolerated. Second treatment can begin at lower temperature and lower again to tolerance.
   c. Bath is given to relieve spasticity; measures to increase heat production should not be used.
   d. Procedure readily adaptable for home use.
   e. All patients do not respond to this treatment, but it is worthy of fair trial.
2. *Preparation*
   a. Explain purposes of the treatment to minimize apprehension and obtain full cooperation of the patient.
   b. Determine and record patient's temperature, pulse, and respiration.
   c. Prepare patient with halter and loincloth or trunks.
3. *Treatment*
   a. Place patient in tank.
   b. Time: 10 to 20 minutes as tolerated.
   c. Remove from tank; dry thoroughly.
   d. Therapeutic exercise follows as tolerated.
4. *Completion of treatment*
   a. Determine and record temperature, pulse, and respiration after treatment.
   b. Treatment temperatures should be recorded for each treatment.
   c. Record treatment response and progress.

References

1. Bassett, S. W.; and Lake, B. M.: "Use of Cold Applications in the Management of Spasticity." *P. T. Review,* 1958 (May), pp. 333-334.
2. Boynton, B. L.; Garramore, P. M.; and Bucz, J. T.: "Observations on the Effects of Cool Baths for Patients With Multiple Sclerosis." *P. T. Review,* 1959 (May), pp. 297-299.

HUBBARD TANK FOR BURNS (Saline Bath)

Effects and indications

1. Cleanse away necrotic tissues.
2. Stimulate healing.
3. Relax and relieve pain.
4. Prepare for exercise to prevent deformities.
5. Prepare for skin grafting.

Equipment

1. The Hubbard tank with water at 94° to 98° F., 12 inches deep, contains about 190 gallons, and at 8 pounds per gallon the water weighs 1,520 pounds.
2. The isotonic saline solution (0.9%) is made by adding sodium chloride (NaCl) 0.9% of 1,520 pounds or 13.68 pounds.
3. Sterile linen as needed.
4. Clean linen as needed: bath towels, washcloths, and compresses.
5. Dressings as needed.
6. Basin and newspaper wrapping for disposal of dressings removed.
7. Halter and loincloth or bath towel to cover the patient as needed.

Procedure for burns

1. *Important considerations*
   a. Watch the patient closely.
   b. Take him out of the tank at any sign of shock.

  c. Check the pulse and respiration.
  d. Avoid drafts—the patient is susceptible to respiratory infection.
  e. Be sure that no dressings are free in the water while turbine is in use as they may clog the drain (a screen may be obtained to use on turbines).
  f. A metal stretcher plinth should be employed if available, or if stretcher canvas is used it should be changed and laundered.

2. *Preparation of patient*
  a. Explain the treatment to minimize the patient's apprehension.
  b. Have all the materials at hand for care of the patient before and after treatment.
  c. Do not leave the patient unattended; have two attendants.
  d. Prepare the patient with a halter and loincloth or as required.
  e. Remove as many dressings as possible without disturbing the burned areas.

3. *Treatment*
  a. With a hoist move the patient to a carrier and lower into the tank; support the head.
  b. Allow the patient to soak long enough to loosen the dressings.
  c. You may or may not use the turbine; it depends on the tolerance of the patient.
  d. Exercises in water depend on the condition of the patient; they are range-of-motion exercises to avoid contractures.
  e. Time: 10 to 30 minutes, depending on the condition of the patient and exercises ordered.
  f. Remove the patient from the tank on a carrier; unburned areas should be dried gently.
  g. In a case involving extensive burns, the patient should be transferred to a carrier covered with a sterile sheet. The patient may be returned to his room for further care or go to surgery for skin grafting.

h. Smaller burn areas may have a dressing applied in the physical therapy department as ordered. This is usually done by a nurse from the floor service in charge of the patient.

i. See that the patient is in good alignment position on the carrier for safe transportation to his room.

4. *Completion of treatment*

a. Keep a record of successive progressive treatment and progress.

b. Wrap and dispose of old dressings.

c. Clean and disinfect the tank thoroughly; may use rubber gloves. "Dreft" is excellent to remove greasy film; washing and rinsing twice takes away burn odors. Run the turbine in "Dreft" solution for cleaning.

References

1. Harmer, B.; and Henderson, V.: *Textbook of the Principles and Practice of Nursing.* New York, Macmillan, 1955, p. 1178.
2. Licht, S.: *Therapeutic Heat.* New Haven, Elizabeth Licht, vol. 2, pp. 221, 377, 378.

HUBBARD TANK FOR DECUBITUS ULCERS (Hub. Tank)

Effects and indications

1. Cleanse away necrotic tissue.
2. Stimulate healing.
3. Relax and relieve pain and discomfort.
4. Prepare for exercise to prevent deformities.
5. Prepare for skin grafting.

Equipment

1. The Hubbard tank with water at 94° to 98° F., 12 inches deep, contains about 190 gallons, and at 8 pounds per gallon the water weighs 1,520.

2. The brine solution is made up as follows:
   a. Sodium chloride (NaCl): 5% of 1,520 pounds, or 76 pounds.
   b. Magnesium sulfate (MgSO₄): 2½% of 1,520 pounds, or 38 pounds.
   c. Clean linen as needed—sheet, bath towels, compresses.
   d. Dressings as needed.
   e. Basin for disposal of dressings.
   f. Halter and loincloth or bath towel to cover patient as needed.

Procedures

1. *Important considerations*
   a. Remove the dressings as much as possible before the treatment.
   b. Be sure no dressings are free in the water while turbine is operating as they will clog the drain (a screen may be obtained to use on Ille turbines).
   c. Skin care after tank treatment is important for intact skin, to keep it in good condition.
   d. The stretcher canvas should be changed and laundered.
2. *Preparation*
   a. Prepare the patient with halter and loincloth as indicated; the patient may be draped with a bath towel over the abdomen and pubic areas to allow adequate exposure of the decubitus areas (coccygeal or trochanteric).
3. *Treatment*
   a. Place the patient in the Hubbard tank with the water temperature at 94° to 98° F.
   b. The turbine may be used, directed carefully at the decubitus areas.
   c. Exercises may be given as directed.
   d. Time: 1 to 30 minutes, depending on condition of the patient and the exercise program.
   e. Remove the patient from tank to a stretcher or treatment

table; dry, taking special care as directed, with dressings for decubitus areas.

f. Keep a record of treatment progress.

g. Observe the special instructions for cleaning of tank.

References

1. Brown, A. F.: *Medical Nursing.* Philadelphia, W. B. Saunders Co., 1957, p. 633.
2. Nyquist, R.: "Brine Bath Treatments for Decubitus Ulcers." *J.A.M.A.,* Feb. 28, 1959, pp. 927-932.

THE RUSSIAN BATH (Russ. B.)

Definition

A body steam bath given with the patient reclining with his head outside of the steam room or cabinet.

Effects and indications

1. Preheating for tonic cold procedures, temp. 110° to 120° F., usually 115° F. (5 to 10 min.).
2. To produce sweating, temp. 110° to 120° F., usually 115° F. (5 to 10 min.).
3. For production of short mild fever therapy.
4. To increase the body temperature (100% humidity, no heat loss).
5. Increase in pulse rate, blood pressure, and metabolism.
6. Marked peripheral vasodilation.
7. Indications: Rheumatoid arthritis, gout, obesity, alcoholism and other addictions.

Equipment

1. Steam room with a slab.
2. Padding and sheet on the slab.

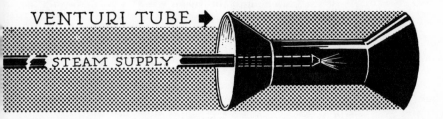

3. Towel for draping around the neck.
4. Air pillow with a cover.
5. Turkish towels for protection of the patient.
6. Material for a hot foot bath and cold compress to the head and neck.
7. Paper cup or glass and straw with a pitcher of drinking water.
8. Drape sheet, shower cap, thong sandals.
9. Ice bag and cover.
10. Fomentation on the slab under the spine.
11. Fomentation may be used in the steam room to wrap the feet.

Procedure

1. *Important considerations*
   a. Contraindicated in hypertension, diabetes, and cardiac impairment.
   b. Check on elimination. The patient should have had a bowel movement within 24 hours previous to treatment time.
   c. Have the patient void before the treatment.
   d. Increased perspiration eliminates some waste; encourage fluid intake.
2. *Preparation*
   a. Prepare the steam room with padding and a sheet.
   b. Drain the steam line.
   c. Place a fomentation for the spine.
3. *Treatment*
   a. Count the pulse, take the temperature.

b. Assist the patient into the steam room, cover him with a Turkish towel.

c. Arrange a drape around the neck, apply a cold compress to the head, give a hot foot bath, apply an ice bag to the heart if the pulse is 80 or above.

d. Remove the foot tub; give water to drink.

e. Turn on the steam gradually. Increase to 110° F., then count time.

f. Count the pulse every 5 minutes.

g. Change the cold compress to the head frequently (cold compress to the neck may be added if necessary).

h. Fluid intake as indicated during treatment.

i. Give a graduated spray or other treatment as ordered.

j. Take the temperature and pulse.

k. Watch for rapid pulse, dizziness, or fainting. Stay with patient.

l. See that patient is adequately cooled.

4. *Completion of treatment*

a. Have the patient rest after the treatment.

b. Report time, pulse, reaction, and temperature.

References

1. Abbott, G. K.; Moor, F. B.; and Nelson, K. J.: *Physical Therapy in Nursing Care.* Washington, D.C., Review and Herald Pub. Assn., 1941, pp. 131-133.
2. Kovacs, R.: *Manual of Physical Therapy.* Philadelphia, Lea and Febiger, 1951, p. 202.
3. Finnerty, G. B.; and Corbitt, T.: *Hydrotherapy.* New York, Frederick Ungar Pub. Co., 1960, pp. 137-140, 142.

MEDICATED RUSSIAN BATH (Med. Russ. B.)

Definition

A general medicated steam bath to the entire body given with the patient reclining and head enclosed.

Effects and indications

1. To relieve inflammation of mucous membranes in common colds and sinusitis.
2. To relieve inflammation and congestion, and to loosen secretions in the tracheo-bronchial tree in acute and chronic bronchitis.

Equipment

1. Steam room with slab.
2. Padding and sheet on slab.
3. Window drape.
4. Air pillow with cover.
5. Turkish towels for draping and protection from condensation of steam if necessary.
6. Material for hot foot bath.
7. Compress or ice bag if needed.
8. Shower cap and thong sandals.
9. Fluids as needed.
10. Fomentation for the spine.
11. Medication for inhalant, 1 ounce.
12. Drape sheet; bath blanket may be needed.

Procedure

1. *Important considerations*
    a. Control steam, increase temperature slowly to provide greater ease of inhalation.
    b. Avoid chilling. Relaxation of the mucous membranes and dilation of peripheral blood vessels increase the danger of chilling.
    c. Avoid moist cold over the sinus areas.
2. *Preparation*
    a. Prepare the steam room with padding and a sheet. Drain steam line.

    b. Place a pillow inside the steam room.

    c. Place a fomentation for the spine.

    d. Protect the hair with a shower cap.

3. *Treatment*

    a. Assist the patient into the steam room and cover him with a Turkish towel.

    b. Give a hot foot bath and fluids to drink.

    c. Add medication to a cloth on the steam supply pipe.

    d. Count the pulse. Apply an ice bag to the heart if pulse is 80 or above.

    e. Place a dry compress over the eyes to avoid irritation.

    f. Remove the foot bath.

    g. Close the steam room, turn on the steam slowly to provide greater ease of inhalation of medicated steam. Check the time.

    h. Temperature 105° F.—not over 110° F.; duration 10 to 15 minutes, usually 10 minutes.

    i. Count the pulse every 5 minutes.

    j. Allow the patient to wait while the steam is reduced.

    k. Give a graduated spray or other treatment as ordered. Wrap the patient with a drape sheet or bath blanket to avoid chilling.

4. *Completion*

    a. Allow the patient to rest before leaving the department since he is very susceptible to cold because of relaxation of mucous membranes and dilation of peripheral blood vessels.

    b. Infrared is sometimes ordered applied to the face in sinusitis after medicated steam.

    c. Report treatment time, pulse, and reaction.

Note: The following formula for medication eliminates the compound tincture of benzoin and is cheaper and cleaner than older formulae: Add 64 grams of camphor gum and 64 grams of natural menthol crystals to 1 gallon of eucalyptus oil.

ELECTRIC LIGHT BATH (E. L. B. or Elb)*

Definition

An application of heat to the body by radiant energy with the patient usually in a sitting position.

Effects and indications

1. As a preheating measure for a tonic procedure to follow (duration 5 to 8 min.); slight increase in temperature, less than 1° F.
2. To produce sweating (duration 5 to 8 min.).
3. Reduction of blood pressure due to marked peripheral vasodilatation.
4. Mild heating for neuroses.
5. Rheumatic conditions.
6. Chronic nephritis.
7. Psychoneurosis.
8. Peripheral neuritis.
9. Obesity.
10. Hypertensive vascular disease.

Equipment

1. Cabinet.
2. Stool.
3. Ice bag with cover.
4. Basin of ice water.
5. Material for hot foot bath.
6. Paper cup and straw.
7. Pitcher of drinking water.
8. Drape sheet and thong sandals.
9. Shower cap if needed.
10. Two hand towels for head turban.

---

*Because the electric light bath is usually accompanied by some hydrotherapeutic procedure, it is included here.

11. TwoTurkish towels for neck drape.
12. Two Turkish towels for stool and floor.

Procedure

1. *Important considerations*
   a. The electric light bath is contraindicated if the patient has diabetes, cardiac impairment, or advanced arteriosclerosis, or is emaciated.
   b. Conversive heating is produced because light energy meets skin resistance; thus heat is generated in the tissues.
   c. To promote elimination, drink water freely.
2. *Preparation for treatment*
   a. Preheat the cabinet.
   b. Drape the patient, take the pulse and respiration.
   c. With the patient seated on a stool give a hot foot bath to tolerance (104° to 110° F.) to hasten reaction and prevent cerebral congestion.
3. *Treatment*
   a. Turn the cabinet lights off and adjust the stool for height.
   b. Cover the stool and floor with towels.
   c. Assist the patient into the cabinet and remove the drape sheet.
   d. Close the door, turn on the lights, caution the patient not to touch the lights.
   e. Apply an ice bag to the heart if the pulse is 80 or above.
   f. Drape a wet Turkish towel around the neck to keep the hot air from rising to the face; apply a turban to head.
   g. Renew the head turban and towel to neck frequently, keep the patient cool.
   h. Give cool water to drink frequently.
   i. Check the pulse and respiration every 5 minutes; if pulse rate rises to 120 or if the patient has dyspnea, stop the treatment.
   j. Note the skin reaction and the amount of perspiration; also, note the general reaction of the patient, watch for signs of dizziness or fainting.

k. Turn off the cabinet lights, wrap the patient in drape sheet to avoid chilling.

l. Give a graduated needle spray or other cooling measure as ordered.

m. Dry the patient thoroughly.

4. *Completion of treatment*

a. Have the patient rest after the treatment, 20 to 30 minutes.

b. Chart the treatment, pulse, respiration, and sweating reaction.

References

1. Abbott, G. K.; Moor, F. B.; and Nelson, K. J.: *Physical Therapy in Nursing Care*. Washington, D.C., Review and Herald Pub. Assn., 1941, pp. 177-179.
2. Bierman, W.; and Licht, S.: *Physical Medicine in General Practice*. New York, Hoeber, 1957, pp. 92, 93.
3. Finnerty, G. B.; and Corbitt, T.: *Hydrotherapy*. New York, Frederick Ungar Pub. Co., 1960, pp. 132-135.
4. Harmer, B.; and Henderson, V.: *Textbook of the Principles and Practice of Nursing*. New York, Macmillan, pp. 674, 675.
5. Kellogg, J. H.: *Rational Hydrotherapy*. Philadelphia, Davis, 1928, pp. 707-711.
6. Licht, S.: *Therapeutic Heat*. New Haven, Elizabeth Licht, 1958, vol. 2, pp. 195-197.
7. Watkins, A. L.: *Electrotherapy*. Philadelphia, Lea and Febiger, 1958, pp. 47, 48.

HOT BLANKET PACK (H. Bl. Pk.)

Definition

The hot blanket pack is an application of moist heat to the whole body by means of multiple fomentations covered by three dry wool blankets and one cotton blanket.

Effects

1. Elevation of body temperature and pulse rate with profuse perspiration.

8—M.H.M.

2. Maximal peripheral vasodilation.
3. Analgesia and muscular relaxation.
4. Increased respiration, with greater elimination of carbon dioxide, resulting in alkalosis.

Indications

1. Selected cases of nephritis, acute or chronic.
2. Eclampsia.
3. Common cold and influenza.
4. Rheumatoid arthritis.
5. Any disease in which vasodilatation and sweating are desirable.
6. Renal or gallstone colic.

Equipment

1. One double wool blanket or 2 single wool blankets.
2. One single wool blanket.
3. Two cotton bath blankets.
4. Twelve fomentations, rolled tightly and placed in a lined foot tub.
5. Basin of ice water.
6. Compress cloths: one hand towel, one wash cloth.
7. Drinking glass with straw or drinking tube.
8. Two Turkish towels.
9. Ice bag.

Procedure

1. *Important considerations*
   a. This kind of hot blanket pack does not have to be hurried since the fomentations hold heat better than a wet blanket.
   b. Have the ice bag handy in case it is needed.
   c. Avoid chilling the patient, especially in the wintertime.
   d. Duration of the blanket pack depends upon effect desired.

2. *Preparation for treatment*
   a. Have the patient void; check bowel elimination.
   b. Check the patient's pulse.
   c. Give the patient a cleansing bath if necessary.

3. *Treatment*
   a. Spread the double blanket on the treatment table, bringing it up to cover the lower half of the pillow.
   b. Now place the fomentations on the blanket, sedative side up, as follows:
      (1) Two across the back.
      (2) One across the hips.
      (3) Two lengthwise for the backs of the thighs and the legs (fold under so the heels do not rest on the fomentation).
   c. Now spread the dry single wool blanket on top of the fomentations; then spread the dry bath blanket in the same manner.
   d. Direct the patient to lie down on his back, so that the blanket rests halfway under the head to allow room for mitering blankets over the shoulders.
   e. Wrap the bath blanket around the patient; then wrap the single dry wool blanket around him.
   f. Place the remaining fomentations on the patient with the hot side down, as follows:
      (1) One across the chest (two if needed).
      (2) One across the abdomen.
      (3) One down the top of each leg (do not let fomentation rest on the toes).
      (4) Place one fomentation around the bottom of the feet on outside of the blanket; now wrap the double blanket snugly around patient and tuck under the feet.
      (5) Place a towel over the wool blanket around the neck.
      (6) Place a folded bath blanket under the knees to prevent hyperextension of knees.

(7) Apply a cold compress to the head and neck when the patient begins to perspire.

(8) Do not leave the patient while in the blanket pack, check the pulse every 5 minutes.

(9) Remove one arm from the pack and give a vigorous cold mitten friction, then the other arm, chest, and abdomen. Now remove pack completely and finish the cold mitten friction to the legs and back.

(10) Cover the patient with a sheet and blanket.

4. *Complete the treatment*

   a. Let the patient rest for 20 minutes or give follow-up treatment as ordered.

   b. Chart the treatment, time, pulse, reaction.

Note: If fomentations are not available refer to procedure for using a blanket in Finnerty and Corbitt, *Hydrotherapy,* 1960, pp. 116-118.

References

1. Abbott, G. K.; Moor, F. B.; and Nelson, K. J.: *Physical Therapy in Nursing Care.* Washington, D.C., Review and Herald Pub. Assn., 1941, p. 137.
2. Finnerty, G. B.; and Corbitt, T.: *Hydrotherapy.* New York, Frederick Ungar Pub. Co., 1960, pp. 116-118.
3. Kellogg, J. H.: *Rational Hydrotherapy.* Philadelphia, Davis, 1928, p. 623.

VARIATIONS OF HOT BLANKET PACK
A. HOT TRUNK PACK (H. Tr. Pk.)

In this pack heat is specifically applied to the trunk area.

Effects and indications

1. This pack is useful for digestive disturbances.
2. Useful in the relief of pain in any form of colic, no cold application being used to conclude the procedure.

Equipment

Equipment is essentially similar to that for the hot blanket pack, except that 5 fomentations only will be needed.

Procedure

Proceed as for the hot blanket pack, placing 2 fomentations lengthwise under the back and the remaining 3 fomentations over the chest, abdomen, and hips. The extremities are not included, but the hot foot bath is given simultaneously. The patient and the foot tub should be covered with the blanket. Apply a cold compress to the head and neck. Duration, 15 to 20 minutes; complete the treatment by giving an alcohol rub with warm alcohol. Avoid chilling. See that the patient is comfortable.

B. HOT HIP AND LEG PACK

In this pack heat is specifically applied to the pelvis and the lower extremities.

Effects and indications

This pack is a most efficient derivative measure and combined with an ice bag over a congested area is useful for depletion of acute inflammation of internal organs, as in pelvic infections, salpingitis, and cellulitis. It is also useful in arthritis with involvement of the hips, knees, and ankles. In this case an ice bag is not needed.

Equipment

Equipment is essentially similar to that for the hot blanket pack.

Procedure

The procedure is done in the same manner as for the hot blanket pack, except that the application of heat is made to the trunk below the waist and to the lower extremities. Apply a cold compress to the head and neck; an ice bag may be applied over the inflamed area as ordered by the physician. To conclude the treatment a cold mitten friction may be given, omitting the area where the ice bag has been applied. Duration, 15 to 20 minutes. In cases of arthritis a hot mitten friction may conclude the treatment. Be sure that the patient does not get chilled. Leave him comfortable.

C. HOT LEG PACK

In this pack the heat is applied below the hips specifically to the feet, legs, and well over the knees.

Effects and indications

This pack can be used for derivative effects but is also an efficient method of treating the nonambulatory arthritic patient.

Equipment

One single wool blanket, one draw sheet, and 5 fomentations will be sufficient for this pack.

Procedure

Place the single wool blanket over the lower end of the treatment table so that one half hangs over the end of the table. Place two fomentations side by side on the blanket lengthwise of the table. Fold the lower end of the blanket over the fomentations and cover with a draw sheet. Place the lower extremities on the draw sheet one on each fomentation and fold the draw sheet from each side over the adjacent extremity and cover from one side with the doubled wool blanket. Over each extremity place one fomentation extending from the thigh to the foot. Do not cover toes or heels. Place the fifth fomentation across bottom of the feet and around up over the extremities. Cover with the doubled blanket from the other side. Keep the head cool with a cold compress. Duration, 15 to 20 minutes. Upon removal of the pack give cool sponging to the extremities. Follow with an alcohol rub to the body. Be sure the patient is comfortable.

WET SHEET PACK (W. Sh. Pk.)

Definition

A wet sheet pack is a procedure in which the patient is wrapped in a wet sheet, outside of which are dry blanket coverings to regulate evaporation and to control the temperature.

Effects

The effects of a wet sheet pack depend upon its duration and number of blankets applied to control evaporation. According to the degree of heat generated within the pack, it passes through three stages as follows:
1. Cooling or evaporating.
2. Neutral.
3. Heating and sweating.

Indications

1. Cooling stage: Antipyretic in fevers.
2. Neutral stage: Insomnia, mania, delirium, restlessness.
3. Heating and sweating stage: Alcoholism, nicotine poisoning, selected cases of chronic nephritis, and gout. It may also be used in transient fevers of infants and children, in bronchitis, common colds, and influenza.

Equipment

1. Material for a hot foot bath.
2. Material for a cold compress.
3. Large double wool blanket (with others as may be needed).

4. Two large sheets.
5. Bucket of cold water 60° to 70° F.
6. One Turkish towel, one hand towel for cold compress.
7. Fomentations, hot-water bottle, or infrared lamp.

Procedure

1. *Important considerations*
   a. The effects of a wet sheet pack are obtained by regulation of evaporation and control of temperature.
   b. The wet sheet pack must come in close contact with the skin in all areas.
   c. Miter dry blankets at neck and shoulder to prevent entrance of air and chilling.
2. *Preparation for treatment*
   a. Have all materials at hand.
   b. Explain procedure to patient.
   c. Give patient hot foot bath ten minutes with cold compress to head (the feet and entire body should be warm).
   d. Have patient void.
3. *Treatment. Note:* The following procedure of wrapping sheet and blankets applies to all stages:
   a. The entire body must be warm before the pack is applied —if not, precede pack with a heating treatment such as electric light bath, hot tub bath, hot spray, or hot foot bath.
   b. Place a double and a single blanket lengthwise on the treatment table. The upper end should cover the lower half of the pillow.
   c. Wring the sheet as dry as possible from cold water and spread it out upon the blanket so that the upper end will be a little below the upper edge of blanket.
   d. The patient then lies down upon the wet sheet with shoulders three or four inches below the upper edge.
   e. Both arms should be raised while one side of the sheet is wrapped quickly around the body. Draw the sheet smoothly in contact with the skin in all places; tuck under on opposite side.

f. Below the hips the sheet is wrapped around the leg on the same side.

g. The arms are then lowered and the opposite side of the sheet is drawn smoothly over body, tucked in, and folded over the shoulders and across the neck.

h. The blanket is now mitered in at the shoulder and neck, the corner tucked under the opposite shoulder. Pull the remainder of the blanket over and tuck under the body and feet.

i. Do the same as above with the other side of the blanket: Miter at the shoulder and neck; tuck under the opposite shoulder, wrapping the rest of the blanket around the legs and feet.

j. Additional blankets may be laid over the patient and tucked in along the sides and about the feet.

k. A Turkish towel is placed about the neck to protect the face and neck from contact with the wool blanket and to exclude air.

l. Duration according to the effect desired—evaporating, neutral, heating, or sweating.

m. Remove the patient from the pack accordingly.

4. *Completion of treatment*

a. Report the treatment duration and results.

b. Have the patient rest after the treatment.

c. Take care of equipment.

References

1. Abbott, G. K.; Moor, F. B.; and Nelson, K. J.: *Physical Therapy in Nursing Care.* Washington, D.C., Review and Herald Pub. Assn., 1941, pp. 142-146.
2. Brown, A. F.: *Medical Nursing.* Philadelphia, W. B. Saunders Co., 1957, p. 697.
3. Harmer, B.; and Henderson, V.: *Textbook of the Principles and Practice of Nursing.* New York, Macmillan, 5th ed., pp. 625-632.
4. Krusen, F. H.: *Physical Medicine.* Philadelphia, W. B. Saunders Co., 1941, pp. 470, 484-485, 491.

◇ ◇ 5 ◇

TECHNIQUE OF
MEDICATED BATHS

MEDICATED BATHS

Saline bath

1. *Solution:* To a full tub (30 gal.) of water at neutral temperature add 8 to 9 lbs. of sodium chloride.
2. *Temperature:* 94° to 98° F.
3. *Time:* 10 to 20 minutes.
4. *Effects:*
    a. As a tonic.
    b. First aid in extensive burns.
Note: The saline bath may have different effects depending on:
    a. Percentage of salt used.
    b. Temperature of the water.
    c. Length of the bath.

Alkaline bath

1. *Solution:* To a full tub (30 gal.) of water add 1 lb. of sodium bicarbonate.
2. *Temperature:* 94° to 98° F.
3. *Time:* 10 to 20 minutes.
4. *Effects:* Allays the irritation of certain drug reactions, eczema, itching, hives, etc.

(110)

Starch bath No. 1

1. *Solution:* Sixteen ounces of dry starch (Linit) to a tub (30 gal.) of water; stir.
2. *Temperature:* 94° to 98° F.
3. *Time:* 20 minutes.
4. *Effect:* Relieves skin irritations. Finish the bath by patting dry, or fanning.

Starch bath No. 2

Same as above except that the starch is boiled until clear, then added to the bath water.

Aveeno bath

1. *Solution:* To a full tub (30 gal.) of water at neutral temperature add one pint (2 cups) Aveeno. (Aveeno is a finely ground oatmeal.)
2. *Temperature:* 96° to 98° F.
3. *Time:* 15 to 30 minutes.
4. *Effect:* Relieves skin irritations.

Note: The Aveeno bath is not as drying as a starch bath. The Aveeno may be put into a coarse muslin bag and soaked in a basin of hot water to avoid lumping. The bag may be used to squeeze the medication into the bath water and to lave the solution gently over areas of the body, such as the shoulders, which are not immersed.

Precipitation of the Aveeno in the water makes the bottom of the tub slippery, so care should be taken to assist the patient out of the tub to prevent his falling.

Potassium permanganate bath

1. *Solution:* To a full tub (30 gal.) of water at neutral temperature add 50 grains (10 5-grain tablets) of potassium permanganate dissolved in one quart of boiling water.
2. *Temperature:* 94° to 98° F.

3. *Time:* 15 to 30 minutes.
4. *Effect:* Antiseptic, astringent, and deodorant.
Note: Potassium permanganate stains linen (old linens might be used).
   a. Dissolve medication in a glass or enamel container as potassium permanganate is corrosive to metal. A tongue blade may be used to stir the solution until dissolved.
   b. The patient's skin will discolor brown. Dry by careful blotting, taking special care of areas which may be denuded or draining.
   c. The tub and the container for the solution should be cleaned with Bon Ami to remove potassium permanganate stains.

Combination alkaline bath

1. *Solution:* To a full tub (30 gal.) of water add 8 ounces of sodium bicarbonate and 8 ounces of dry starch.
2. *Temperature:* 94° to 98° F.
3. *Time:* 10 to 20 minutes.
4. *Effect:* Soothes irritated skin.

Sulfur bath

1. *Solution:* From ½ to 1 ounce of potassium sulfate is dissolved in a small quantity of hot water and added to 15 gallons of water.
2. *Temperature:* 90° to 102° F.
3. *Time:* 10 to 20 minutes.
4. *Effect:* Given for acne, and other skin diseases, such as scabies. Dry without friction.
Note: A mixture of bensyl benzoate, DDT, benzocaine, and an emulsifier is perhaps more often used at present for scabies.

Balpine bath (pine needle oil)

1. *Solution:* To a full tub of neutral water, add ½ ounce of "Balpine oil."

2. *Temperature:* 96° to 98° F.
3. *Effect:*
   a. Sedative.
   b. Refreshing.
   c. Produces a slight hyperemia of the skin.

Alpha Keri (water-dispersible oil)

1. *Solution:* One to two tablespoonfuls of Alpha Keri (4 to 6 capsules) to a tub of water.
2. *Temperature:* 94° to 98° F.
3. *Time:* 15 to 20 minutes.
4. *Effect:* Antipruritic.

Oil of cade (oil of juniper)

1. *Solution:* Two to four tablets of Almay tar to a full tub of water.
2. *Temperature:* 94° to 100° F.
3. *Time:* 15 to 20 minutes.
4. *Effect:* Antipruritic.

References

1. Brown, A. F.: *Medical Nursing.* Philadelphia, W. B. Saunders Co., 1957, pp. 474, 695.
2. Finnerty, G. B.; and Corbitt, T.: *Hydrotherapy.* New York, Frederick Ungar Pub. Co., 1960, pp. 154-158.
3. Harmer, B.; and Henderson, V.: *Textbook of the Principles and Practice of Nursing.* New York, Macmillan, 1957, 5th ed., pp. 619, 623, 624.

6

UNDERWATER AND SPA THERAPY

UNDERWATER THERAPY

For many centuries water has been used therapeutically, for its chemical, thermal, or mechanical effects. Not until the twentieth century have its hydrostatic and hydrodynamic properties, specific gravity, molecular cohesion, and buoyancy been utilized in the treatment of disease. In 1924, Lowman and Roen[1] worked out definite underwater treatment procedures. About the same time Dr. Lowman's presentation of a film on the techniques of underwater exercise at the American Orthopedic Association meeting in Atlanta, Georgia, stimulated interest in pool therapy.

President Franklin D. Roosevelt's use of the Warm Springs, Georgia, resort drew the attention of the general public to the usefulness of underwater treatments.

According to Kolb[2], water is an exercise medium in its own right. The values of pool therapy depend to a large extent upon the therapist's skill and his understanding of the physical forces which operate in water. Intimately associated with the therapist's ability is the physician's knowledge of indications for pool therapy. Lowman[3] maintains that the physician should inquire into the facilities available and, further, that the cooperation between the physician and therapist should be very close, for the better the cooperation the better will be the results.

Values

One of the major values of underwater therapy is the opportunity it provides of treating the patient safely and at an earlier date than would otherwise be possible, particularly in orthopedic cases. This results in improved morale. Because the warmth of the water has a sedative effect, neurotic patients and those with increased muscular tension show improvement. Cerebral congestion is relieved because of the dilation of the peripheral blood vessels. Many compensation cases can be mobilized easily, an economic factor which should not be overlooked. Pool therapy is also valuable in meeting the exercise requirements and improving function in the rehabilitation patient. Avoidance of the pain-spasm-pain cycle and its inhibitory psychic reaction is, in the opinion of Lowman[3], an important reason for beginning exercises early with water as the medium.

Prescription of pool therapy

The prescription should include the diagnosis, the physiological response desired, and the frequency and duration of the treatment. Lowman's[3] recommendations are as follows:

Neuromuscular cases treated most frequently are: (1) postsurgical—plastic surgery to muscles, tendons, and joints; (2) posttraumatic—primarily injury to back and knees; (3) arthritides and postural deviation, in the order given. Pool treatments are of major value for postsurgical leg and hip procedures, such as shelf operations for congenital dislocation of the hip, cup arthroplasties, prosthetic hips, osteotomies, and fractures of the femur repaired by various methods of pinning or grafting.

Physical principles

The effect of water temperature in treatment is frequently mentioned, but there are other physical principles which should be given consideration. These are the forces of hydrostatic pressure, density, the movement of the body, buoyancy, and cohesive forces, commonly known as viscosity.

The effect of hydrostatic pressure depends upon the depth to which the body is submerged, for the greater the depth, the greater will be the pressure which is exerted. *Density* also influences pressure, for as density increases so does pressure. If the body is at rest, the pressure is the same in all directions beneath the surface of the liquid, and the total force exerted on the submerged body is equal to the pressure per unit area multiplied by the total area of the body.

The *buoyancy*, or lifting effect of a liquid, known as Archimedes' principle, may be stated in two different ways. An immersed body is buoyed up by a force equal to the weight of the liquid which it displaces. Or, it may be said that the immersed body seems to lose weight and this apparent weightlessness is equal to the weight of the water which is displaced. Because of this principle, an individual weighing 100 pounds out of water will weigh less than five pounds when nearly submerged in the water. The individual walking in water bears only the weight of the portion of the body which is above the water as a result of this buoyancy effect.

Buoyancy supports the part so that the muscles are able to act more freely and have only viscosity and other physical forces to overcome. The buoyancy of each part of the body and the body as a whole will depend upon the postural alignment, since this influences the amount of the body surface subjected to the lifting force. Buoyancy is influenced by the weight of the bones in relation to the muscles, the amount and distribution of fatty tissue, and the depth and expansion of the chest, according to Kolb[2]. The law of flotation states that a body which is floating displaces its own weight of the liquid in which it floats.

The *viscosity*, or cohesive force within the body of water, will give slight resistance to underwater movement in any direction. This is the only significant force encountered in motion parallel to the surface. It should be borne in mind that if salt water is used, the hydrostatic force and buoyancy will be increased because of the greater weight of the water.

As an object moves through water it encounters resistance or hydrodynamic force. It can be readily understood that the more rapidly an object moves through water, the greater will be the hydrodynamic force that must be overcome. However, this is not in simple proportion, but the force required to move through the water will increase at a rate which is out of proportion to the increased motion.

Hydrodynamic force is also related to the size and the form of the object moving through the water. A small, streamlined object will have less force acting upon it than a larger object of irregular shape. It must be remembered that this force is active in any plane of movement.

Specific gravity is the ratio of the weight of a given volume of a substance to that of an equal volume of water. A substance with a specific gravity of less than 1 will float. The specific gravity of the human body is slightly less than 1.

PLANNING AND CONSTRUCTION FOR POOL THERAPY

Preliminary Planning

Before the construction of a therapeutic pool is undertaken, a survey of the community need should be conducted. Pools are expensive to construct and maintain, and require a large amount of space which might be more advantageously used if other medical facilities in the area can provide adequately for this type of therapy.

Area and placement of the pool

Considerable thought should be given to the organization of the pool area. Its location in relation to the rest of the physical therapy department is important. It should permit free flow of traffic to corridors and elevators for easy transportation by wheelchair and stretcher. It should be so situated that maximum supervision is possible by a qualified physical therapist.

9—M.H.M.

Supply room

A centrally located area for warmed sheets and towels and for drying the patient must be provided. Storage space for equipment used in the pool will be necessary. Provision will need to be made for the drying and sterilization of swimming suits and trunks. The psychological importance of privacy should not be forgotten. There must be a satisfactory method for the disposal of wet linen.

Dressing rooms, showers, and toilets

Staff dressing rooms, toilets, and showers should be conveniently adjacent to the pool. Separate showers and toilets for patients should also be placed near the pool. The showers should be large enough to care for nonambulatory patients as well as those who are able to shower themselves. Use of a spray for stretcher patients is often preferred to the overhead shower. Taking a shower before and after therapy in the pool is usually the recommended procedure.

Doorways for showers and toilets must be wide enough to permit easy movement of stretchers and wheelchairs. Space must be provided on one side of the pool to permit safe handling of patients without unnecessary strain and discomfort of the staff.

Floor surfaces

Nonskid tile is the preferred floor surface for ease of care and safety, although smooth concrete has often been employed. Corrugated rubber mats are used in small pool areas to prevent slipping.

Lighting and ventilation

Adequate indirect lighting should be provided. If possible, daylight should be utilized; glare, however, should be minimized. The pool area should be well-aired, but free of drafts. Finnerty and Corbitt[4] suggest that air conditioning can be utilized to handle the heat and excessive humidity.

Physical aspects of the pool

Pool sizes vary according to the need. The smallest recommended size is 10 x 12 feet, but 15 x 24 or 15 x 30 feet seems to meet the needs of the average facility more adequately. A depth of 4 feet 6 inches or 5 feet is considered satisfactory for the deep end, with a depth of 2 feet 6 inches at the shallow end. While a very slight slope may be necessary for adequate drainage and cleaning, the floor of the pool should be practically flat, so that the disadvantage of walking on a slant is not added to the patient's disability or inability to walk. Different graduation of levels in the form of steps will be found more useful for ambulation activities and for placing underwater chairs or plinths. Care should be taken that the transition from one level to the next is clearly marked by different colored tile, so that the levels are clearly discernible. A guardrail may be necessary to prevent patients from getting into the deeper areas unawares.

Equipment

Rust-resistant handrails around the sides of the pool at water level are recommended. Chrome, bronze, and nickel are some of the metals employed. Lowman[3] suggests that these be 1½ inches in diameter. Similar railings should be provided on both sides of the steps leading into the pool.

Parallel bars should be so positioned that free movement is possible on every side, with the bars being 10 or 12 inches below the surface of the water. Weighted chairs or stools, rubber cushions, cork floats, wooden paddles, weighted boots and crutches, rubber hand and foot flippers, weighted plinths, balls and floating toys, clip-on canvas slings to fit the bars for free use of arms and legs, are examples of equipment which is necessary for good pool therapy. Licht[5] recommends the Lowman plinth as the one best designed for underwater use. Adequate support is given to the trunk, and handholds are provided. Intelligent and constant care of equipment used in pools is essential, or rapid deterioration will take place.

Water

A therapeutic pool must have adequate provision for disinfection and filtration of the water. A twice-daily analysis of chlorine content is usually required by public-health authorities; this can be done by the hospital engineer. Weekly samples of water should be taken for bacterial testing. The pool should either be cleaned by vacuum or emptied and cleaned every one to six weeks, depending on the size of the pool and its usage. Floor areas and wooden steps, if used, should be cleaned daily to prevent cross infection by dematophytes.

Water temperature depends upon the condition to be treated. A temperature of 98° to 100° F. is recommended by Licht[5] and also by Bolton and Goodwin[6] for spastic paralysis, while 92° to 95° F. is considered adequate when exercise is the primary objective. If active swimming is to be used therapeutically, temperatures of 85° to 90° F. are suitable. Due consideration should be given to the objectives of treatment. There is little heat loss from the body even at 90° F. If the pool is too warm, fatigue and heat exhaustion may occur.

Indications

In addition to the recommendations by Lowman[3] which have already been presented, the following conditions respond well to underwater therapy: muscle weakness, such as seen in peripheral nerve lesions, poliomyelitis, polyneuronitis, rheumatoid arthritis, cerebral palsy, torticollis, postural deviations, postencephalitis, fibrositis, congenital neurological defects, preprosthetic stump preparation, paraplegia, and psychiatric conditions.

Length of treatment

Treatment time may vary from 5 minutes in the beginning to 30 minutes. In psychiatric cases, pool therapy is recommended for 1 to 2½ hours. The first treatment may consist of gradual immersion only. Basic safety measures should be taught, such as relaxation in the water, breath control, and prone and supine floating recoveries. A recovery is considered adequate for the patient if he is able to get his head out of the water and maintain this position until help can reach him.

Contraindications

Therapy in a pool is contraindicated in any febrile condition. Licht[5] recommends a normal temperature for 72 hours before treatment is instituted. Underwater therapy is contraindicated in cardiac decompensation, very high or very low blood pressure, acute inflammation of joints or active joint disease, acute painful neuritis, nephritis or kidney infection, acute systemic infections, infections of the eye, ear, nose, or throat, active pulmonary tuberculosis, acute poliomyelitis, infective skin conditions. Treatment in the pool is not recommended during menstruation or for incontinent patients. Underwater therapy for the incontinent is usually done in the Hubbard tank. Following therapy, if the patient should have symptoms of undue fatigue or loss of appetite, pool therapy should be discontinued.

For positioning and technique, the reader is referred to the excellent manual by Lowman and Roen[1] entitled *Therapeutic Use of Pools and Tanks.*

Exercise progression

Kolb[2] has summarized activities to be considered in the pool and the principles underlying progression. The easiest exercises should be done first. The hydrostatic forces operating in various planes are listed below:

1. "Active-assistive movement in any plane."
2. "Movement from below toward the surface to the buoyant level of the part. The dominant force of buoyancy will be assisting."

3. "Joint motion parallel to the surface of the water at the buoyant level. Only the molecular forces within the liquid are significant since the part is weightless at the buoyant level."
4. "Movement from the buoyant level toward the surface. In addition to the molecular forces the weight of the superimposed liquid increases the difficulty level."
5. "Movement downward from the buoyant level. The dominant force of buoyancy offers more resistance."
6. "Movement downward from the buoyant level utilizing floats to increase the buoyant force."

Kolb reminds us that steps two and four in this series have restricted usefulness, since the range of motion for many movements is limited.

Summary

In summary, it can be said that while the therapeutic pool requires considerable space in the hospital and is expensive to maintain, it is a very useful therapeutic tool in the hands of experienced physical therapists under the direction of a physician who understands its value and limitations. Its usefulness is limited largely to orthopedic and neurological conditions, although therapeutic swimming has been found useful in the treatment of psychiatric patients.

References

1. Lowman, C. L.; and Roen, S. G.: *Therapeutic Use of Pools and Tanks.* Philadelphia and London, W. B. Saunders Co., 1952.
2. Kolb, M. E.: "Principles of Underwater Exercise." *Phys. Ther. Rev.* 37:361 (June), 1957.
3. Lowman, C. L.: "Therapeutic Indications for Pool Therapy." *Phys. Ther. Rev.* 37:324 (April), 1957.
4. Finnerty, G. B.; and Corbitt, T: *Hydrotherapy.* New York, Frederick Ungar Pub. Co., 1960.
5. Licht, S.: *Therapeutic Exercise.* New Haven, Elizabeth Licht, pp. 280-289.
6. Bolton, E.; and Goodwin, D.: *An Introduction to Pool Exercises.* Edinburgh and London, E. and S. Livingstone, Ltd., 1956.

SPAS AND HEALTH RESORTS

The term "spa" comes from the name of the town of Spa in the province of Liége, Belgium, where mineral springs were first discovered in 1326. Some 20,000 persons visit this resort annually. A spa is a health resort or watering place possessing a source of mineral water. Spas are found in many parts of the world but are most popular in Europe and especially in Germany. There are over 200 major spas in the German Federal Republic. These are visited annually by hundreds of thousands of persons.

Spas and health resorts have never been developed in the United States as extensively as in Europe but there are several well-known spas in this country: Hot Springs, Arkansas; Saratoga Springs, New York; Clifton Springs, New York; Marlin, Texas; White Sulphur Springs, West Virginia; French Lick Springs, Indiana; and Hot Springs, Virginia.

There are several factors which have retarded the development of health resorts in this country. In Europe most of the spas receive governmental support, but less than ten in the United States receive subsidies from Federal, state, or municipal governments. There is little or no instruction concerning spa therapy in our medical schools, and as a result the American medical profession is not acquainted with it. There are, in fact, few reliable sources of information regarding spas and health resorts. Only a very few American spas have medical supervision, and the operation of others is by laymen or irregular practitioners. The result is that all spa therapy is unjustly regarded by some physicians as quackery.

Spas may be conveniently classified as thermal, saline, gaseous, and iron-bearing. Thermal waters come to the surface at varying temperatures, some so hot that they must be cooled before they can be tolerated and some at cool or comfortable temperatures. Saline waters contain chlorides, sulfates, and carbonates of sodium, potassium, calcium, magnesium, or other elements, usually as mixtures. Gaseous waters contain natural gases under pressure. These are partially discharged when they reach the surface. The common gases are carbon dioxide, hydrogen sulfide, and radon. Iron-bearing waters must contain at least 10 mg. of iron per liter to be so classified.

In addition to mineral water, many spas also employ hot peloids, or muds, classified as: (1) mineral muds or fango, containing volcanic ash, (2) mineral sea muds containing shells of sea animals, (3) organic muds or peat made up of decomposed vegetable matter. These various muds are used as a means of applying moist heat to the surface of the body.

The beneficial effects of spa therapy depend not only on the mineral water but also on the climatic conditions, the restful spa atmosphere, and freedom from responsibility. A prominent feature of the large European spas is the "kurpark," a beautifully landscaped area around or adjacent to the spa for the recreation and enjoyment of the patrons. The location of the spa will determine its climate and the type of diseases for which it is best suited. Some spas have elaborate facilities for amusement such as concerts, theatricals, and other exciting features, which are usually frowned upon by the spa physicians.

Whether the mineral water found at spas has any effects beyond those of fresh water at comparable temperatures is a matter of some controversy. It can be readily conceded, however, that a highly mineralized water would have a higher specific gravity and greater buoyancy effect than fresh water, thus making it superior for underwater exercise. This buoyancy effect varies between 3 and 11 percent of the body weight according to the specific gravity of the medium.

The hydrostatic pressure exerted by mineral water is somewhat greater than that exerted by fresh water. Upon immersion this causes compression of the veins and lymphatics and accelerates venous and lymph flow and even has some hastening effect upon the arterial flow. Hydrostatic pressure also reduces the intra-abdominal and intrathoracic capacity, further accelerating the blood flow toward the heart, whose stroke and minute volume have been observed to increase as much as 24 percent.

German spa physicians maintain that minerals such as iron,

manganese, and copper in ionic form pass through the skin and accomplish a "transmineralization" of the body. There seems to be no one in this country who subscribes to this view. According to McClellan[1], CO_2, hydrogen sulfide, and radon are absorbed through the skin from waters containing these gases.

Patrons of spas frequently drink the mineral water as well as applying it externally. The effects of drinking mineral waters will vary somewhat according to mineral salts contained and their concentration. Mineral waters containing sulfates and phosphates of magnesium, sodium, and potassium are laxative. Some minerals such as iron, iodine, and calcium may be retained in the body and add to its stores of these elements.

Mineral waters may also be inhaled in nebulized form for their soothing effect on the mucosa of the respiratory tract and to facilitate the absorption of gases, especially radon. It is claimed by the German physicians that ten times as much radon is absorbed by inhalation as through the skin. Inhalations of nebulized mineral water are used chiefly for the treatment of chronic respiratory diseases.

There is need for research study of the physiological effects of spa therapy by scientists well qualified for such projects. Among physicians who have observed and have experienced spa treatment, there is no doubt as to its value, but, unfortunately, little or no real scientific evaluation has been done. Within recent years some very fine research institutes have been established at some of the German spas, but personnel to operate them has been in short supply.

A large percentage of persons who seek relief at spas are afflicted with the rheumatic diseases, both articular and muscular. For these conditions hot mineral water containing sulfur has the best reputation. Mud and peat baths, which are available at many spas, are also helpful. Entire dependence should not be placed on the spa therapy, but it should be only one feature of a complete therapeutic program in which proper nutrition and indicated medical treatment should be components. This is true in rheumatoid arthritis, degenerative joint disease, and gout.

Spa therapy is of great value in functional nervous disorders in patients who complain of anxiety, insomnia, tension headaches, and fatigue. Removed from stresses of the home environment to the quiet atmosphere of the spa, with mineral baths and rest, these patients usually do well. Organic nervous diseases needing underwater exercise can also be well handled at properly equipped spas.

Selected cardiovascular patients respond well to the spa regimen. They usually do best at spas where the water is heavily charged with CO_2, which lowers arterial tension and relieves some of the heart's burden. These cases should usually have accompanying massage and carefully supervised graduated exercise.

Such respiratory conditions as chronic sinusitis, pharyngitis, laryngitis, bronchitis, and asthma frequently benefit from spa therapy. For treatment of these conditions nebulized alkaline mineral water is most helpful.

For some gastrointestinal conditions the laxative properties of the mineral waters containing sulfates and phosphates of magnesium and sodium may be of considerable value when taken internally. The chronic "dyspeptic" who habitually overeats will also respond well to the drinking of this type of mineral water.

Other conditions often benefited by the spa regimen are certain skin diseases, especially eczema and psoriasis, obesity, convalescence from prolonged illness, and iron-deficiency anemia. In each of these diseases the proper spa should be selected and other indicated therapy employed.

Reference

McClellan, W. S.: *Spa Therapy in Medical Physics.* Otto Glasser, Year Book Publishers, Inc., Chicago, 1944.

SECTION II

MASSAGE

7

THE RATIONALE
OF MASSAGE

INTRODUCTION

Massage may be defined as the manipulation of the tissues of the body for therapeutic purposes. The word itself is taken from a root meaning "to knead" or "to handle."

Massage is an ancient remedy used both by man and animals. Animals instinctively lick their wounds, cleansing and massaging at the same time. Man has doubtless used massage of a simple type from prehistoric times. It is known to have been employed anciently in China and India. It was described by Homer in 1200 B.C. and by Hippocrates in 460 B.C. It was used in the Greek and Roman baths. In more recent times it was developed to a high degree by Ling of Sweden and Mezger of Holland. Later advocates were Weir Mitchell and Kellogg in the United States, and Cyriax and Mennell in England.

MASSAGE MOVEMENTS

The common movements used in massage are: (1) stroking (effleurage), (2) kneading (petrissage), (3) friction, (4) percussion (tapotment), (5) vibration.

Stroking may be superficial or deep. Superficial stroking con-

sists of long, light, rhythmical stroking movements in which the
effect is reflex in nature. Deep stroking is much heavier, is usually centripetal, and is aimed primarily at emptying veins and
lymphatics by mechanical pressure. Kneading consists in grasping the muscle, picking it up, rolling, and squeezing it according
to the contour of the muscle mass. Kneading is always applied
across the muscle. The muscle should never be pinched with
the tips of the fingers.

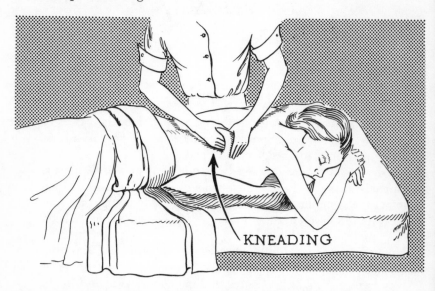

KNEADING

Friction is a deep circular movement in which the fingers do
not glide over the skin but the skin moves with the fingers. It is
not a rubbing motion as the name might suggest. It is intended
to loosen superficial scar tissue or adhesions and break up fibro-
sitic nodules in the muscles and connective tissues. (See picture
on next page.)

Percussion movements consist of clapping, tapping, slapping,
or beating the tissue being massaged. Percussion is one of the
less important massage movements. Vibration is a vibratory or
shaking impulse imparted to the patient's tissues by a continuous

vibration of the operator's shoulder, arm, hand, and fingers. This is a difficult movement which is tiring to the operator and is of questionable therapeutic value. It is rarely employed.

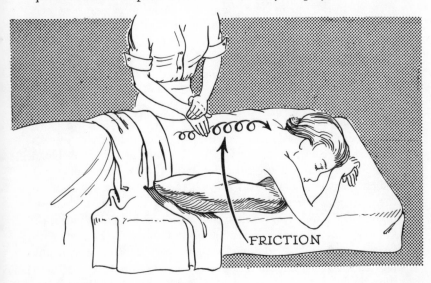

FRICTION

PHYSIOLOGICAL EFFECTS

Circulatory effects

In presenting circulatory effects of massage, we shall consider both the blood and the lymph flow. In the first place, an auto-massage effect on the circulation is produced by the respiratory movements and the contractions of the skeletal muscles. This effect accelerates the propulsion of venous blood back toward the heart. This is so important that prolonged immobilization of the lower extremities slows the venous blood flow to the point where intravenous clotting not infrequently occurs. Such a clot may break loose and travel through the venous system and heart to the lungs as a pulmonary embolus, a very dangerous complication in both medical and surgical patients.

Some of the findings of different investigators on the influence of massage on blood flow have been contradictory. Pemberton and Scull[1] in 1944 reported that massage caused a definite increase in the rate of blood flow. They gave as evidence redness of the skin, an increased skin temperature, and, microscopically, an increased number of functioning skin capillaries. These effects they considered to be partially reflex and partially due to the release in the tissues of histamine and acetylcholine. Clark (quoted by Pemberton) observed increased blood flow and increased sticking and migration of leukocytes through vessel walls following massage.

Wakim et al[2] in a study of the effects of massage in human subjects were unable to confirm the findings of others on blood flow. These authors used the venous occlusion plethysmograph which measures total blood flow, both deep and superficial, in the extremity tested. In normal subjects, patients with rheumatoid arthritis and those with spastic paralysis showed no increase in blood flow following deep stroking and kneading. Patients with flaccid paralysis showed a moderate but consistent increase in the rate of blood flow. The findings of Pemberton and Scull and those of Wakim et al appear to disagree, but not necessarily so, because the former were observing only the superficial circulation while the latter were measuring the total circulation in the extremity.

When we consider the lymph flow, we find general agreement among investigators that massage does increase lymph flow. Bauer et al[3] found that massage hastened the removal of egg albumen from the joints of dogs as measured in the lymph drainage. McMaster[4] demonstrated increased lymph flow after massage, by an intradermally injected dye. Kottke et al[5] compared the influence of massage, passive exercise, and electrical muscle stimulation on lymph flow. All of these caused increased flow, but massage was by far the most effective.

On the blood itself, Mitchell[6] in 1894 in a clinical study found that general massage caused an immediate and marked rise in the number of red blood cells but a lesser increase in hemoglobin. In anemic patients, the increase was maintained about one hour and then gradually returned to the previous level. However, with successive treatments, the increase was longer maintained. These findings of Mitchell[6] were confirmed by Pemberton and Scull[1].

In summarizing the effects of massage on the blood and circulation, we may conclude that massage does increase the superficial blood flow, but probably not the flow to muscles and other deep tissues except in the presence of flaccid paralysis. Lymph flow is definitely increased. General massage causes an immediate increase in the red blood cell count and hemoglobin which is transient but has a tendency to be more prolonged with repetition.

Neuromuscular effects

Pemberton and Scull[1] observed that massage produces muscular relaxation in patients with muscle twitching and spasm. This is common knowledge with physiatrists and physical therapists who deal frequently with this problem. In fibrositis with its accompanying muscle spasm, heat and massage are standard treatment.

In the treatment of muscle atrophy following peripheral nerve damage in cats, massage, according to Suskind *et al*[7], causes a slight retardation of weight loss and definite maintenance of strength in denervated muscle. In dogs Kosman *et al*[8] were unable to observe either a retardation of denervation atrophy or the maintenance of muscle strength. Regardless of whether or not strength and muscle mass are retained, the writer is of the opinion that massage of paralyzed muscle, whether the paralysis is due to an upper or lower motor neuron lesion, does help to maintain muscle in better condition pending restoration of neuromuscular function, if that is eventually possible. This means especially keeping the muscle supple and free from fibrosis.

In some cases of spasticity, massage may not be feasible because of the extreme irritability of the neuromuscular mecha-

nism. However, it may be facilitated by the preliminary application of heat or cold, whichever proves to be the more effective.
In these cases massage must be exceedingly gentle in order to
avoid spasm.

Metabolic effects

Cajori et al[9] and Pemberton and Scull[1] reported that massage,
especially massage to the abdomen, caused diuresis. This diuresis
is accompanied by increased excretion of nitrogen, inorganic
phosphorus, and sodium chloride. There was no effect on crea-
tine or creatinine excretion.

Culbertson[10] observed a decrease in the excretion of nitrogen,
sulfur, and phosphorus in fracture patients receiving massage,
indicating an increased utilization of these elements in tissue
repair. Unlike exercise, massage does not increase oxygen con-
sumption nor does it cause lactic acid production or acidosis.

Kalb[11] reported in 1944 a clinical study of 40 patients afflicted
with obesity and treated with massage. He found that massage
had no effect either on generalized obesity or on local deposits of
fat.

Mechanical vibration

There are many mechanical vibrators on the market for the
public and some also for the use of the medical profession. Some
are for use as hand vibrators, some vibrating pillows, and some
vibrating chairs or beds. Those for professional use in the treatment of patients are the hand-operated type. Although mechanical vibration is not a substitute for manual massage, it does
exhibit some of the effects of massage. It is incorrect to call it
"massage" or, as one concern calls it, "cyclomassage."

Ebel and Wisham[12] reported a study of the effect of mechanical vibration with one of the widely advertised vibrators sold to
the general public. They determined the effect of the vibration
on skin temperature, muscle temperature, and radioactive sodium
clearance from skin and muscle. The average increase in skin

temperature in one series of experiments after 30 minutes of vibration was 2.2° C.; in muscle, the average increase in temperature was an insignificant 0.27° C. The rate of sodium clearance was increased an average of 69 percent from the skin. The rate of sodium clearance from muscle was not significant.

Mechanical vibration may be useful occasionally when manual massage is not available or as a supplement to manual massage. It is not a satisfactory substitute for massage performed by the operator's hands.

INDICATIONS FOR MASSAGE

The prescription for massage should be based on its physiological effects and the pathological condition for which it is given. Based on these considerations, it has many uses. The following are the common indications for massage:

Musculoskeletal conditions

1. Osteoarthritis and rheumatoid arthritis.
2. Myositis, fibrositis, and fibromyositis.
3. Posttraumatic conditions such as sprains, strains, and contusions.
4. Postfracture care.
5. Muscle cramps, including writer's cramp.
6. Torticollis.
7. Amputation stumps.
8. Coccygodynia by the intrarectal method of Thiele[13].

Cardiovascular conditions

1. Cardiac edema.
2. Intermittent claudication of peripheral vascular disease.

Neurological conditions

1. Hemiplegia.
2. Poliomyelitis.

3. Multiple sclerosis.
4. Parkinson's disease.
5. Functional nervous disease.
6. Bell's palsy and other peripheral nerve lesions.

Miscellaneous conditions

1. General massage for secondary anemias.
2. Abdominal massage for constipation.

CONTRAINDICATIONS

There are some diseases in which massage should never be used because of the danger of spread of the disease to neighboring or distant tissues. The following is a list of the common contraindications:

1. Known or suspected benign or malignant new growths. Massage of a malignant tumor would be likely to cause metastasis through the blood or lymph circulation.
2. Acute phlebitis, thrombophlebitis, or phlebothrombosis. In these diseases, massage over the involved vein might dislodge a blood clot or embolus which would lodge in the lung, causing infarction and possibly death.
3. Lymphangitis is an infection which would be spread by massage.
4. Acute inflammatory conditions of the skin, soft tissues, joints, or bones would be made worse by massage.
5. Skin diseases such as eczema, acne, furuncles, ulcerations, and wounds should obviously not be massaged.
6. Hyperesthesia of the skin may render massage too painful to tolerate.
7. Acute communicable disease would not ordinarily be benefited by massage and the operator would be in danger of contracting the disease and communicating it to others.
8. Pregnancy is a contraindication for abdominal massage.

GENERAL CONSIDERATIONS

Massage is seldom prescribed alone, but is usually part of a complete prescription written by the physician according to his estimate of the patient's needs. It is usually preceded by some form of heat for its relaxing and analgesic effect. The best form of heat to produce relaxation of muscle is moist heat in the form of fomentations or immersion baths. Infrared radiation or ultrasound are second choices but are effective. Diathermy, although the heat of choice for some conditions, is not a good muscle relaxer. The paraffin bath is the most satisfactory form of heat for the hands of patients with rheumatoid arthritis; it is a very satisfactory preparation for massage. If exercise is indicated in the individual case, it is usually given following massage.

Massage should be given in a warm, quiet room. The patient should be placed in the most comfortable position possible on a firm table of proper height for the most effective treatment. Massage should never be attempted over the patient's clothing. The hands of the masseur should be kept free from calluses and roughness. The patient's skin is usually lubricated with a massage cream or oil or dusted with powder. These are removed at the end of the treatment.

The general type and dosage of massage should be indicated in the physician's prescription. However, in the administration of massage, much must be left to the judgment and experience of the masseur. The treatment should be long enough to be effective, and yet the patient should not be fatigued. The duration of massage to a local area may vary from 5 to 15 minutes. General massage may last 45 minutes to an hour. Frequency of treatment may range from daily to twice weekly. The dosage and frequency of massage is based entirely on the individual patient's condition as judged by the attending physician.

References

1. Pemberton, R.; and Scull, C. W.: *Massage (Medical Physics)*. Chicago, Yearbook Publishers Inc., 1944.

2. Wakim, K. G.; Martin, G. M.; Terrier, J. C.; Elkins, E. C.; and Krusen, F. H.: "The Effects of Massage on the Circulation in Normal and Paralyzed Extremities." *Arch. Phys. Med.* 30:135 (March), 1949.

3. Bauer, W.; Short, C. L.; and Bennett, G. A.: "The Manner of Removal of Proteins From Normal Joints." *J. Exper. Med.* 57:419, 1933.

4. McMaster, P.: "Changes in the Cutaneous Lymphatics of Human Beings and in Lymph Flow Under Normal and Pathological Conditions." *J. Exper. Med.* 6:347, 1937.

5. Ladd, M. P.; Kottke, F. J.; and Blanchard, R. S.: "Studies on the Effect of Massage on the Flow of Lymph From the Foreleg of the Dog." *Arch. Phys. Med.* 33:604 (Oct.), 1952.

6. Mitchell, G. K.: "The Effect of Massage on the Number and Hemoglobin Value of Red Blood Cells." *Am. J. Med. Sc.* 107:502, 1894.

7. Suskind, M. J.; Hajek, M. M.; and Hines, H. M.: "Effects of Massage on Denervated Muscle." *Arch. Phys. Med.* 27:133 (March) 1946.

8. Kosman, A. J.; Wood, E. C.; and Osborne, S. L.: "Effect of Massage Upon the Denervated Skeletal Muscle of the Dog." *Arch. Phys. Med.* 29:489 (Aug.), 1948.

9. Cajori, F. A.; Crouter, C. Y.; and Pemberton, R.: "The Physiologic Effect of Massage." *Arch. Int. Med.* 39:281, 1927.

10. Culbertson, D. P.: "Certain Effects of Massage on the Metabolism of Convalescing Fracture Cases." *Quart. J. Med.* 1:401, 1932.

11. Kalb, S. W.: "The Fallacy of Massage in the Treatment of Obesity." *J. Med. Soc. New Jersey* 41:407 (Nov.), 1944.

12. Ebel, A.; and Wisham, L. H.: "Effect of Massage on Muscle Temperature and Radiosodium Clearance." *Arch. Phys. Med.* 33:399 (July), 1952.

13. Thiele, G. H.: "Coccygodynia and Pain in the Superior Gluteal Region." *J.A.M.A.* 109:1271 (Oct. 10), 1937.

◇ ◇ 8 ◇

Technique of MASSAGE

CENTRIPETAL RUB (C. R. or Cpr.)

Centripetal rub consists of four movements.

1. Lubricating.
2. Stroking—*centripetal*—deep, firm.
4. Stroking—*centrifugal*.
3. Percussion—if indicated.

Purpose

The centripetal rub (Cpr.) may be used as a sedative massage with deep stroking (or effleurage) as the principal movement, or for general treatment following general applications of hydrotherapy for tonic purposes.

Upper extremity

1. Lubricate from the wrist to the shoulder two times, coming down to the fingers with four rotary movements.
2. *Stroking—centripetal*
   a. *Deltoid*—support the upper arm at the elbow medially. Stroke the deltoid up and over the shoulder to the subclavian area below the clavicle—use the lateral hand over the anterior deltoid three times and over the lateral and posterior deltoid three times.
   b. *Biceps and triceps*—support the patient's arm at the elbow

(139)

with the hands alternating while stroking the biceps to the axilla, and the triceps over the shoulder three times each. (*Note:* The biceps and triceps may each be done three times separately.)

c. *Elbow*—support the arm at the wrist laterally—stroke the medial aspect of the elbow (antecubital fossa) three times.

d. *Forearm*—support the forearm (with the elbow resting on the table) at the wrist, to stroke the forearm medially and laterally (flexors and extensors) three times each. (*Note:* These muscle groups may each be done three times separately, supporting the forearm at the wrist with the opposite hand.)

e. *Hand*—support the hand by grasping as if shaking the hand. Stroke the back of the hand and up over the wrist three times. Turning the hand over, palm up, stroke the inside of the hand three times.

f. Deep firm stroking from the hand to the shoulder, alternating the medial and lateral surfaces three times each. Glide back without breaking contact with the skin.

3. *Percussion* (only if indicated)

Spatting from the wrist to the shoulder up and down once.

4. *Stroking—centrifugal* (light sedative)

With both hands on the shoulder stroke down the arm to the fingertips three times.

Lower extremity

1. *Lubricate* from the ankle to the hip, coming down to the foot with six to eight rotary movements.

2. *Stroking—centripetal*

a. *Thigh*—with two hands give firm, even stroking from the knee to the hip (anterior superior spine) three times.

(1) Anterior.

(2) Medial and lateral.

(3) Posterior (to gluteal fold).

b. *Knee*—use both hands simultaneously, medially and laterally (the thumbs at side of the patella and the fingers at the popliteal area) to give firm, even stroking three times. Extend the movement from well below to well above the joint.

   c. *Leg* (knee extended)
      (1) With both hands stroke the anterior surface starting at the ankle, posterior to the malleoli. (Glide back without breaking contact with the skin three times.)
      (2) Support the knee in an outward rotation. Use the other hand to give firm, even stroking to the calf muscles from the ankle to the knee three times.

   d. *Foot* (knee extended)
      (1) *Dorsum and sides*—with both hands stroke the dorsum of the foot three times. Give firm, even pressure with the fingers to the sides of the foot. Use the thenar surface of the hand on the middorsum area.
      (2) *Sole*—support the foot at the ankle and stroke with the medial hand three times, giving a reinforced stroke to the heel each time.

   e. Deep stroking from the foot to the hip three times (knee extended). With two hands stroke the anterior surface medially and laterally; then stroke the posterior surface to the gluteal fold.

3. *Percussion* (only if indicated). Roll the leg in inward rotation to give spatting laterally from the ankle to the hip and return once.

4. *Stroking—centrifugal* (light sedative)
With both hands at the hip stroke lightly the medial and lateral surfaces to the toes three times.

Chest (supine position)

The patient should be in a position of relaxation—slight flexion at the knees to relax the abdominal muscles, a pillow for the head (avoiding too much flexion) to relax the muscles of the neck, and positioning of the arms to relax the pectoral muscles. Drape the patient as needed.

1. *Lubricate*

   Stroking from midline (sternum) to the shoulders, make rotary movements on the shoulder and upper chest. Then circle the breast area, making rotary movements on the ribs two times.

2. *Stroking—centripetal* (deep firm)

   a. *Neck*—place the hands at the sides of the neck with the fingers at the mastoid area—use the heel and palm of the hand to stroke down each side toward the sternum three times. *Note:* Avoid heavy pressure over the clavicle; also avoid pressure with the thumbs over the throat.

   b. *Pectorals*—place one hand on each shoulder—using the heel of the hand, stroke from the insertion of the pectorals at the humerus in and down to the sternum three times.

   c. *Lower pectorals and serratus anterior*—place the hands with the thumbs at the lower sternum—stroke under the breast area out and up to the axilla. Strokes should be progressively lower to cover the serratus anterior and the rib cage three times.

3. *Percussion*

   No percussion movements are applied to the chest.

4. *Reflex stroking* (light sedative)

   With one hand on each shoulder stroke in and down over the pectorals to the lower sternum—continue with stroking out and up to the axilla three times.

Abdomen (Supine position)

The patient should be positioned in the same manner as for the chest procedures. Drape the patient carefully, using a Turkish towel to cover the chest area, tucking it under securely at each side. The sheet covering the lower extremities should be folded down at the lower abdomen and tucked securely under each hip.

1. *Lubricate*

   Place the hands with the thumbs at the midline and make rotary movements to cover the abdominal area.

2. *Stroking—centripetal* (deep firm)
   a. Using both hands—one hand each side of the midline—stroke downward simultaneously toward the hips three times.
   b. Place the hands at the midline to stroke the upper area of the abdomen outward and downward following the direction of the lower ribs. For the middle area stroke from the median line outward toward the bed line, and for the lower area make the strokes downward and outward in the direction of the hip joints. Do each part one or two times.
3. *Percussion*
   No percussion movements are applied to the abdomen.
4. *Reflex stroking* (light sedative)
   Place one hand on each side of the midline at waistline. Stroke downward simultaneously toward the hips three times.

Back (prone position)

Use a pillow under the lower chest and abdomen and a small pillow or a folded towel for the head.
1. *Lubricate*
   Stroke up the spine and return, making rotary movements to the shoulders, scapulae, ribs, waist, and buttocks two times.
2. *Stroking—centripetal*
   a. Spine and outer back.
      (1) With both hands give firm pressure up each side of the spine to the neck. Gliding laterally out over the trapezius, return without pressure to the base of the spine three times.
      (2) With both hands give firm pressure on the outer lateral areas, stroking up over the ribs and shoulders, glide back down the spine to return three times.
   b. *Trapezius*
      (1) With both hands stroke the upper trapezius from the ear to the shoulder (bilaterally) three times.
      (2) With both hands stroke the middle trapezius from the base of the neck to the acromion process three times.

(3) With both hands stroke the lower trapezius from the spine at the lower angle of the scapula to the acromion process three times.

(4) *Note:* The trapezius may be done unilaterally with an alternating two-hand count of four repeated two or three times.

c. *Latissimus dorsi*

(1) With both hands (the thumbs lateral to the spine) begin at the waistline—stroke from the spine out and up to the axillae—turn to use the heel of the hand on the posterior axilla and the deltoid three times.

(2) Beginning with the hands between the angle of the scapulae and the waistline, stroke out to the axillae three times as in (1).

d. *Buttocks*

(1) With both hands (begin below the hips on each side) stroke the gluteal area up to the lumbosacral area. Cross over and continue stroking laterally over the iliac crest (with pressure applied by the heel of the hand) three times.

e. *Spine and outer back*

(1) Repeat firm pressure up each side of the spine with both hands three times.

(2) Repeat firm pressure with both hands up the outer lateral area from the waist up over the ribs and shoulders, gliding back down the middle to return three times.

3. *Percussion* (only if indicated)

Give spatting up the outer side of the back, returning down the medial area lateral to the spine. Do the far side of the back first, then the near side in the same manner.

4. *Stroking—centrifugal* (light sedative)

a. Stroke the outer back with both hands from the shoulders to the hips two or three times.

b. Stroke down the spine from the neck with the hands alternating three times each.

GENERAL MASSAGE

Upper extremity (supine position)

1. *Lubricate*—stroking from the wrist to the shoulder; coming down to the fingers with four rotary movements two times to cover the skin surface.
2. *Stroking—centripetal* (deep firm)
    a. *Deltoid*—support the upper arm at the elbow medially. Stroke up and over the anterior deltoid to the subclavian area below the clavicle three times. Stroke over the middle and posterior deltoid over the acromion process three times.
    b. *Biceps and triceps*—support the patient's arm at the elbow with the hands alternating while stroking the biceps from the elbow to the axilla and the triceps from the elbow up over the shoulder three times each.
    c. *Elbow*—support the arm at the wrist laterally—stroke medial aspect of the elbow (antecubital fossa) three times.
    d. *Forearm*—supporting the forearm at the wrist—alternately stroke the flexors (medially) and the extensors (laterally) three times each. *Note:* These muscle groups may each be done unilaterally three times each.
    e. *Hand*—support the hand by grasping as if shaking the hand. Stroke the back of the hand and up over the wrist three times. Turning the hand over (palm up), stroke inside of the hand and down over the wrist three times.
3. *Kneading*
    a. *Shoulder* (deltoid area)
        (1) Support the elbow medially. Give one-hand kneading to the anterior deltoid three times and to the middle and posterior deltoid three times.
        (2) Two-hand kneading to the entire deltoid area down and up three times.
        (3) Follow kneading with deep firm stroking over the anterior, middle, and posterior deltoid up over the shoulder three times.

b. *Upper arm* (biceps and triceps)
   (1) Support the elbow with the arm in position of internal rotation. Give one-hand kneading (beginning at the elbow) to the biceps and the triceps alternately or unilaterally three times each.
   (2) Follow with deep firm stroking from the elbow to the shoulder alternating or unilaterally as kneading was done.
c. *Elbow*
   (1) Support the elbow in position as for upper arm. Give finger and/or thumb kneading (deep friction) to the joint area.
   (2) Follow with deep stroking.
d. *Forearm*
   (1) Support the forearm at the wrist for one-hand kneading of the flexors and extensors from the insertion to the origin at the humeral condyles. The flexor and extensor groups may be done alternately three times or unilaterally three times each.
   (2) Follow with deep stroking alternately or unilaterally three times.
e. *Hand and wrist*
   (1) *Fingers* (the hand should be supported at the wrist and the palm). Each finger is manipulated with a combined stroking and friction movement from the distal phalanx to the metacarpophalangeal joint, one or two times and return; the thumb is also included.
   (2) *Hand*
      (a) Support the palm with the fingertips to give alternate thumb kneading to dorsal interossei spaces (metacarpophalangeal joints to the wrist) once.
      (b) Supporting the hand with the palm up, give alternate or simultaneous kneading of the thenar and hypothenar muscles.
   (3) *Wrist*
      Supporting the hand, give thumb kneading to the

carpal area (radial to ulnar border and return) one or
two times—do the volar and dorsal surfaces.

(4) Follow with deep stroking to the dorsum of the hand
over the wrist and to the palmar surface up over the
wrist.

4. *Entire extremity*—deep stroking from the hand to the shoulder, alternating medial and lateral muscle groups two times
each.

5. *Percussion* (only if indicated)—spatting from the wrist to the
shoulder up and down once.

6. *Reflex stroking* (light sedative)—with both hands on the
shoulder stroke down the arm to fingertips three times.

Lower extremity (supine position)

1. *Lubricate*—stroking up the extremity to the anterior superior
spine of the ilium; return, making rotary movements covering
anterior and posterior, medial and lateral surfaces of the limb
two times.

2. *Stroking—centripetal* (deep firm)
   a. *Thigh*—with both hands give firm even stroking from the
   knee to the hip (anterior superior spine) three times,
   anterior, medial, lateral, and posterior to the gluteal fold.
   b. *Knee*—use both hands simultaneously medial and lateral
   (thumbs at side of the patella and fingers at the popliteal
   area) to give firm even stroking three times. Extend the
   movement from well below to well above the joint three
   times.
   c. *Lower leg* (leg extended)
      (1) With both hands stroke the anterior surface, starting
      at the ankle posterior to the malleoli up to the knee
      three times. *Note:* Do not rub on the shinbone.
      (2) Support the knee with one hand and turn in slight
      outward or inward rotation position of the leg. Use
      the other hand to give firm even stroking to the calf
      muscles from the insertion to the origin three times.

d. *Foot* (leg extended)
  (1) Dorsum and sides—with both hands stroke the dorsum of the foot, including the ankle, three times. Give firm, even pressure with the fingers to the medial and lateral surfaces around the malleoli, using thenar surface of the hand on the middorsal area up front of the ankle.
  (2) *Sole*—support the foot at the ankle and stroke three times, giving additional rotary pressure to the heel with the thenar surface of the hand.

3. *Kneading*
  a. *Thigh*
    (1) With one hand supporting the extremity at the knee, give one-hand kneading to the anterior thigh (quadriceps—insertion to origin) three times.
    (2) Supporting the knee, give one-hand kneading to the medial surface (adductors) three times.
    (3) Supporting the knee, give one-hand kneading to the lateral surface from the knee up over the hip three times.
    (4) With both hands give two-hand kneading (alternating) to the medial and lateral hamstrings from the knee to the gluteal fold.
    (5) Using both hands, give firm even stroking from the knee to the hip three times, anterior, medial, lateral, and posterior (to gluteal fold).
    (6) Two-hand kneading may be given to the anterior thigh (quadriceps, insertion to origin), thoroughly manipulating the vastus medialis and lateralis as well as the rectus femoris.
    (7) Follow with two-hand stroking (deep firm) from the knee to the hip three times.
  b. *Knee*
    (1) With one hand supporting the knee give finger kneading medially and laterally to the joint.
    (2) Giving support under the knee with the fingers, use

the thumbs to give kneading bilaterally around the patella. Thumb kneading may be given to the medial and lateral joint areas simultaneously or unilaterally.

(3) Two-hand kneading (alternating medially and laterally), starting below and working up above the knee joint three times.

(4) Firm even stroking—use both hands simultaneously (medial and lateral), the thumbs at the side of the patella and the fingers at the popliteal area three times.

c. *Lower leg* (extended, with a small pillow under the knee)

(1) Support the leg at the ankle with one hand while giving one-hand kneading to the muscles lateral to the tibia from the ankle to the knee three times.

(2) Support the knee in slight outward rotation. Use the other hand to knead the calf muscles from the ankle to the knee three times.

(3) Two-hand kneading may be given to the calf muscles.

(4) Follow with firm, even stroking from the ankle to the popliteal area three times.

d. *Foot and ankle* (leg extended)

(1) Supporting the metatarsal arch with the fingers, give alternate thumb stroking to the toes.

(2) With the same position give thumb kneading to the metatarsal joint area from the first to the fifth and return.

(3) With the same position give thumb kneading to the dorsal interossei spaces from the toes to the ankle once each.

(4) Grasping the foot with both hands, give two-hand kneading, alternating bilaterally.

(5) Give finger kneading to the ankle bilaterally (anterior and posterior to malleoli).

(6) With both hands stroke the dorsum of the foot, including the ankle, three times.

(7) Support the foot at the ankle—give firm stroking to

the sole of the foot with rotary pressure to the heel three times.

3. *Entire extremity*

Deep stroking from the foot to the hip with both hands three times. (On the thigh, stroke the anterior surface with stroke one, medial and lateral surfaces with stroke two, and the posterior surface [hamstrings] with stroke three.)

4. *Percussion* (only if indicated)

Spatting from the ankle to the hip up and down once.

5. *Reflex stroking*

With both hands at the hip stroke down to the toes three times.

Chest (supine position)

The patient should be in a position of relaxation—slight flexion at the knees to relax the abdominal muscles, a pillow for the head (avoiding too much flexion) to relax the muscles of the neck, and positioning of the arms to relax the pectoral muscles. Drape.

1. *Lubricate*

Stroking from the midline (sternum) to the shoulders, make rotary movements on the shoulder and the upper chest. Then circle the breast area, making rotary movements on the ribs two times.

2. *Stroking—centripetal* (deep firm)

a. *Neck*—place the hands at each side of the neck, with the fingers at the mastoid area; use the heel and the palm of the hand to stroke down each side toward the sternum three times. *Note:* Avoid heavy pressure over the clavicle; also avoid pressure with the thumb over the throat.

b. *Pectorals*—place one hand on each shoulder; using the heel of the hand, stroke from the insertion of the pectorals at the humerus in and down to the sternum three times.

c. *Lower pectorals and serratus anterior*—place the hands with the thumbs at the lower sternum; stroke under the breast area out and up to the axilla. Strokes should be progressively lower, to cover the serratus anterior and the rib cage three times.

3. *Kneading*

Because it is difficult to do kneading, these muscles are manipulated by rolling movements effected by the flat of the hand pressed firmly upon the tissues, first on the pectorals working from the shoulders to the sternum and then on the lower chest from the lower sternum working out and up toward the axilla three times. Kneading may also be done with the thumb and fingers, taking care to avoid pinching. This is followed by the deep stroking movements to the upper and lower chest three times.

4. *Percussion*

No percussion movements are applied to the chest.

5. *Reflex stroking* (light sedative)

With one hand on each shoulder stroke in and down over the pectorals to the lower sternum; continue with stroking out and up to the axilla three times.

Abdomen (supine position)

The patient should be positioned in the same manner as for the chest procedures. It is very important for the knees to be in a flexed position in order to relax the abdominal muscles. Drape the patient carefully, using a Turkish towel to cover the chest area, tucking it securely under at each side. The sheet covering the lower extremities should be folded down at the lower abdomen and tucked in securely under each hip.

1. *Lubricate*

Place the hands with the thumbs at midline and make rotary movements simultaneously to cover the abdominal area.

2. *Stroking—centripetal* (deep firm)

   a. Using both hands, one hand each side of the midline, stroke downward simultaneously toward the hips three times.

   b. Place the hands at the midline to stroke the upper area of the abdomen outward and downward, following the direction of the lower ribs. For the middle area, stroke from the median line outward toward the bedline, and for the lower area make strokes downward and outward directing movement toward the hip joints. Do each part one or two times.

3. *Kneading*

    a. Two-hand alternate kneading to the right side of the abdomen over the ascending colon, up and down three times. Follow the two-hand kneading of the left side of the abdomen over the descending colon three times.

    b. Mass kneading (entire abdominal area), according to Kellogg, is of value when the abdominal wall is considerably relaxed. This is done with two hands.

    c. These movements may be followed by a one-hand maneuver making moderate pressure along the colon: Use the thumb and thenar surface of the hand to make pressure upward over the ascending colon to the hepatic flexure, then transfer pressure to the four fingers over the transverse colon area toward the left (splenic flexure). Finally, using the ulnar border of the palm and hypothenar area, give pressure downward over the descending colon to the sigmoid flexure. This maneuver should be a slow, continuous movement and may be repeated three times. Avoid any pressure over the urinary bladder area.

    d. Follow with deep stroking to the upper, middle, and lower areas of the abdomen.

4. *Percussion*

No percussion movements should be given without specific orders from the physician.

5. *Reflex stroking* (light sedative)

Stroke downward simultaneously three times.

Back

Prone position with a pillow under the abdomen to avoid a lordotic position. A small pillow or folded bath towel may be used for head support.

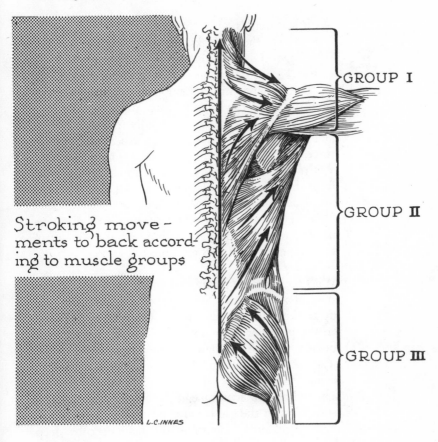

Stroking move-
ments to back accord-
ing to muscle groups

GROUP I

GROUP II

GROUP III

L.C.INNES

1. *Lubricate*
   Stroke up the spine bilaterally; make rotary movements to the
      shoulders, ribs, waist, and hips two times.
2. *Stroking—centripetal* (deep firm)
   a. *Spine and outer back*
      (1) With one hand at each side of the spine, give firm
          pressure up each side of the spine from the lumbo-
          sacral area to the neck. Gliding out laterally over the
          trapezius, return without pressure to the base of the
          spine three times.

    (2) With both hands, give firm pressure beginning at the hip up over the buttocks, ribs, and shoulders. Glide back down the spine to return three times.

  b. Trapezius

    (1) With both hands stroke the upper trapezius bilaterally from the ear to the shoulder three times.

    (2) With both hands stroke the middle trapezius bilaterally from the base of the neck to the acromion process three times.

    (3) With both hands stroke the lower trapezius bilaterally from the spine at the lower angle of the scapulae to to the acromion process three times.

    (4) *Note:* The trapezius may be done unilaterally from the origin to the insertion with an alternate count of four, repeated two or three times.

  c. Latissimus dorsi

    (1) With both hands (thumbs lateral to the spine), begin at lumbosacral area. Stroke from the spine out and up to the axilla, turning to use the heel of the hand on the posterior axilla and deltoid three times.

    (2) Beginning with the hands at the lower angle of the scapulae, stroke out and up to the posterior axilla and deltoid three times.

  d. Buttocks—with both hands begin below the hip on each side, stroking over the gluteal area bilaterally up and in to the lumbosacral area. Continue the maneuver by deep stroking laterally over the iliac crest (with pressure applied by the heel of the hand) three times.

3. *Kneading*

  a. Trapezius

    (1) One-hand kneading of the trapezius upper, middle, and lower fibers unilaterally.

    (2) Two-hand kneading to the upper, middle, and lower sections of the trapezius right and left.

    (3) Follow with deep stroking bilaterally upper, middle, and lower fibers three times.

b. *Latissimus dorsi*
   (1) One-hand kneading—beginning below the scapula up laterally to the posterior axilla unilaterally right and left.
   (2) Two-hand kneading unilaterally right and left.
   (3) Follow with deep stroking bilaterally from the lumbosacral area up and out to the posterior axilla and the deltoid three times.

c. *Buttocks*
   (1) One-hand kneading—beginning below the hip up and medialward to the lumbosacral area unilaterally right and left.
   (2) Two-hand kneading unilaterally right and left.
   (3) Follow with deep stroking bilaterally from the hip to the lumbosacral area. Continue the maneuver laterally along the iliac crest three times.

d. *Entire back*
   (1) Two-hand kneading—beginning at lower back, do the lateral area up to the shoulder. Return medially lateral to spine, right and left sides, three times.
   (2) Follow with deep stroking to the spine and outer back bilaterally three times.

e. *Spine*
   (1) Digital stroking down the spine reinforced three times. Use the index and the third finger (one on each side of the vertebrae).
   (2) Finger kneading or "skin rolling" up the spine over spinous processes of the vertebrae with forefingers over the advancing thumbs, using hands bilaterally.
   (3) Muscle grasping (finger kneading) with the hands alternating up and down the spine. (The thumbs on one side and the fingers on the other side of the spine.)
   (4) Digital circular friction up each side of the spine with one hand reinforced by the other. This may also be done by using the thumbs alternating bilaterally.

   (5) Digital kneading down the spine; longitudinal to-and-fro movement at the vertebral interspaces bilaterally with the index and second fingers reinforced.

   (6) Follow with digital stroking down the spine (reinforced).

  f. Entire back (additional maneuvers)

   (1) Palmar kneading to the shoulders at medial, lateral, and inferior angles of the scapulae three times. Rotation of the scapulae may be included.

   (2) Deep stroking to the latissimus dorsi bilaterally from the lumbosacral area to the posterior axillae; endeavor to stretch low back musculature with this maneuver.

   (3) Deep stroking to the buttocks three times. Beginning at the hips, stroke up and in to the lumbosacral area. Continue laterally along iliac crest (with pressure applied by heel of the hand) three times.

   (4) Transverse wringing—beginning at the lower back, with one hand each side, traverse horizontally across the back with pressure toward the midline, alternating right and left. Progress upward to the shoulders and return down to the hips once.

4. *Stroking—centripetal* (deep firm)

 a. Spine and outer back

   (1) Firm, deep pressure up each side of the spine from the lumbosacral area to the neck three times.

   (2) With both hands beginning at the hips, stroke up over the buttocks, ribs, and shoulders. Glide back down the spine to return three times.

5. *Percussion* (only if indicated)

 Spatting up each side laterally and down medially (avoid the spine).

6. *Reflex stroking—centrifugal* (light sedative)

 a. Outer back, shoulders to the hips with two hands three times.

 b. Spine, one-hand stroking, alternating, from the neck to sacrum.

APPENDIX

PRESCRIPTION-WRITING ABBREVIATIONS

1. Anatomical Abbreviations

Abd.	Abdomen
Bk.	Back
Ch.	Chest
Fing.	Finger
Ft.	Foot
H.	Hand
Hd.	Head
Hp.	Hip
Musc.	Muscle
Lg.	Leg
Lt.	Left
Nk.	Neck
Rt.	Right
Sh.	Shoulder
Sp.	Spine
Tr.	Trunk

2. Procedure Abbreviations

Alc. R.	Alcohol rub
Chem. Pk.	Chemical pack (hydrocollator)
C. Comp.	Cold compress
C. M. F. or Cmf.	Cold mitten friction
C. R. or Cpr.	Centripetal rub
C. Z.	Cold sitz bath
Cont. B.	Contrast bath
Cont. B. Arms and H.	Contrast bath, arms and hands
Cont. B. Ft. and Lg.	Contrast bath, feet and legs

(157)

E. L. B. or Elb. . . . . Electric light bath
Evap. W. S. Pk. . . . . Evaporation wet sheet pack
Fo. . . . . Fomentations
Grad. B. . . . . Graduated bath
Grad. Spr. . . . . Graduated spray
Heat. Comp. . . . . . . Heating compress
Heat. W. S. Pk. . . . . . Heating wet sheet pack
Heat. Tr. Pk. . . . . . Heating trunk pack
H. Bl. Pk. . . . . Hot blanket pack
H. & C. Arm B. . . . Alternate hot and cold arm bath
H. & C. Ch. . . . . Alternate hot and cold to the chest
H. & C. Douche . . . . Contrast douche
H. &. C. Hd. . . . Alternate hot and cold to the head
H. & C. Lg. B. . . . . Alternate hot and cold leg bath
H. & C. Perc. D. . . Alternate hot and cold percussion douche
H. & C. Z. . . . . . Alternate hot and cold sitz bath
H. Comp. . . . . Hot compress
H. Douche . . . . . . Hot percussion douche
H. Ft. B. or Hft. B. . . . . . . Hot foot bath
H. Lg. B. . . . . Hot leg bath
H. Spr. . . . . Hot spray
H. Tr. Pk. . . . . Hot trunk pack
H. T. B. . . . . Hot tub bath
Hub. Tank . . . . Hubbard tank
Ice Pk. . . . . Ice pack
KMnO₄ B. . . . . . Potassium permanganate bath
Med. Russ. B. . . . . . Medicated Russian bath
M. A. B. . . . . Moist abdominal binder
Neut. B. . . . . Neutral tub bath
Neut. Douche . . . . . . Neutral douche
Par. B. . . . . Paraffin bath
Perc. D. . . . . Percussion douche
Russ. B. . . . . Russian bath
S. Gl. or Sgl. . . . . Salt glow
Spr. . . . . Spray
Sweat. W. S. Pk. . . . . . Sweating wet sheet pack

Tub B.   .   .   .   .   Tub bath
W. Sh. Pk.   .   .   .   .   Wet sheet pack
Wpl. B.   .   .   .   .   Whirlpool bath
Z. B.   .   .   .   .   Sitz bath

CLEANING PREPARATIONS

1. Med-I-Solv (XC-300), organic acid detergent made by Klenzade Products, Inc., Beloit, Wisconsin.
2. HC-8, a chlorinated cleanser, made by Klenzade Products, Inc., Beloit, Wisconsin. HC-8 is sold in 100-pound barrels.
3. Heteraphyl 100% detergent, sold by Columbia Wax Company, Riverdale Drive, Glendale, California. Use 1½ ounces to 1 gallon of water.
4. Ben Hur detergent by Colgate. May be used for cleaning tanks. Rinse well.
5. Wescodyne "Tamed Iodine," from West Chemical Products, Inc., 42–16 West Street, Long Island City 1, New York.
6. pHisoHex—Winthrop Laboratories, New York 18, New York.

ORIGINAL CLEANUP

Wash all surfaces of the tanks with Med-I-Solv (XC-300).
1. Apply 1 to 2 oz. Med-I-Solv to wet a nylon-enclosed cellulose sponge.
2. Scrub all surfaces of the tank and pump shafts.
3. Rinse thoroughly.
4. Repeat on areas where heavy deposits were not removed.

MAINTENANCE BETWEEN USAGES

Whirlpools

Wash all surfaces of the tank with HC-8 (powdered chlorinated cleanser by Klenzade).

1. Rinse the tank thoroughly with hot water.
2. *a.* Fill a plastic bucket with hot water.
   b. Add 2 oz. HC-8 to each gallon.
   c. Place the bucket under the shaft of the motor.
   d. Lower the shaft into the bucket and operate the motor on and off.
   Note: Run the motor only long enough to get the solution circulated, or excess foaming will occur.
3. Pour the solution into the bottom of the tank.
4. Thoroughly scrub all the surfaces.
5. Drain and rinse.

Large tanks

1. Rinse the tank thoroughly with hot water.
2. Add 2 oz. HC-8 to 1 gallon of hot water in a plastic bucket.
3. Scrub all the surfaces thoroughly; rinse.
4. Drain and rinse again.

SUPPLIES FOR DAILY MAINTENANCE

1. HC-8 (powdered chlorinated cleanser by Klenzade).
2. Hose with the spray nozzle (pressure gun handle).
3. Long-handle brush (nylon).
4. pHisoHex (antibacterial action—used on patient).
5. Wescodyne "Tamed Iodine" (germicide).

FINAL CLEANUP AT END OF WEEK

Wash all surfaces of the equipment following chlorinated cleanup with Med-I-Solv (XC-300).
1. Add Med-I-Solv, 1 to 2 oz., to 1 gallon of hot water.
2. Follow the same procedures with this solution as followed with the chlorinated cleaner.

INDEX

Cajori, F. A. 134
Camphorated oil, in heating compress
    to throat 48
Cancer, hyperthermia for 22
Capillary pressure in local heated
    areas 6
Cardiac edema, massage for 135
Cardiovascular patients, spa therapy
    for 126
Carter, R., and Moor, F. B. 8
Cellulitis, hot hip and leg pack for 105
Central nervous exhaustion, cold
    mitten friction for 63
Centripetal rub massage 139-144
Cerebral palsy, Hubbard tank for 84
    underwater therapy for 120
Cerebrovascular accidents, cold wet
    pack for 23
Chemical pack (hydrocollator) 32-34
    for muscle spasm 32
    for relief of pain 32
    to increase blood flow 32
Chest congestion, hot foot bath for 37
Chest pack, heating 48, 49
    for chronic bronchitis 48
    for pneumonia 48
    for whooping cough 48
Chloramphenicol, for typhoid fever
    22
Claudication (intermittent) of periph-
    eral vascular disease, massage
    for 135
Cleaning preparations 159
Cleansing tub bath 78, 79
Cleanup, final, at end of week 161
    original 159
Coccygodynia, massage for 135
Cohesive forces (viscosity) 115, 116
Cold, for spasticity 22, 23
    general applications of 21-25
    local application of 7-9
    analgesic effect of 7, 8
    in refrigeration anesthesia 8
Cold, common, foot bath for 37
    hot blanket pack for 102
    sinus congestion from, treatment
    of 18
    wet sheet pack for 107
Cold mitten friction 63, 64
    compared with salt glow 65
    for central nervous exhaustion 63
    for convalescence after fevers 63
    for hyperthyroidism 63
    for hypochromic anemia 63

for paralysis agitans 63
to produce reaction effect 24
Combination alkaline bath 112
Compress, cold 44-46
    for congestion 44
    for pain due to edema or trauma
    44
    use of, in application of hot and
    cold to head 56, 57
    heating 46-49
    applied to joints, for joint pain
    and inflammation in rheumatic
    fever, chronic arthritis, or
    synovitis 48
    applied to throat, for pharyngitis,
    tonsillitis, laryngitis 48
    for pain of sore throat or rheu-
    matic joints 46
Conduction of heat 5, 19
Congenital neurological defects,
    underwater therapy for 120
Congestion, cold compress for 44
    chest cold, hot and cold to chest
    for 58
Consensual (reflex) effects of applica-
    tion of heat or cold 9, 10
Constipation, abdominal bandage for
    49
    abdominal massage for 136
Contrast bath 17-19, 53-55
    for congestive headache 53
    for fractures 53
    for impaired venous circulation
    53
    for indolent ulcers 53
    for indurative edema 53
    for lymphangitis 53
    for rheumatoid arthritis 53, 54
    for sprains, strains, and contusions
    53
    immersion periods of 18, 19
Contrast douche 77
Contrast local applications 51, 52
    for local injuries with ecchymosis
    (contusions) 51
    for pain from trauma or strain 51
    for wound infections 51
Contusions, contrast bath for 53
    massage for 135
Convalescence, after fevers, cold mit-
    ten friction for 63
    from prolonged illness, spa therapy
    for 126
Convection of heat 5, 19

Joint disease, degenerative, spa
    therapy for 125
Joint inflammation, of rheumatic
    fever, ice pack for 50
Joint pain, acute, treatment of 8
Judgment, place of, in treatment
    vii, viii

Kalb, S. W. 134
Kellogg, J. H. 43, 44
Kenny pack, application of, to extrem-
    ities 7
Kneading (petrissage) in massage
    129, 130
Kolb, M. E. 114, 121, 122
Kosman, A. J. 133
Kottke, F. J. 132
Krusen, E. M., Wakim, K. G. 7
Krusen, F. H. 20
Kuntz, A. 11, 12
Kymograph, use of, in test of cutaneo-
    visceral reflexes 14

Landis, E. M. 6
Landis, E. M., and Gibbon, J. H. 12
Laryngitis, heating compress for 48
    spa therapy for 126
Latent heat, of fusion 3
    of vaporization of water 3
Leukocytosis, stimulation of, by
    application of moist heat 20,
    29
    as defense against disease 20
Levine, M. G. 22, 23
Licht, S. 119, 121
Local heated areas, capillary pressure
    in 6
Lowman, C. L. 115, 119, 120
Lowman, C. L., and Roen, S. G. 114,
    121
Lymphangitis, contrast bath for 53
Lymph flow as affected by massage
    132

McClellan, W. S. 125
McCutcheon, M. 20
McMaster, P. 132
Mackenzie, J. 10
Maintenance, between usages 159,
    160
    of large tanks 160
    supplies for daily 160
Mania, full immersion bath for 81
    wet sheet pack for 107

Massage, art requiring diligent prac-
    tice vii
  centripetal rub 139-144
    four movements of 139
    of abdomen 142, 143
    of back 143, 144
    of chest 141, 142
    of lower extremity 140, 141
    of upper extremity 139, 140
  circulatory effects of 131-133
  contraindications 136
  effleurage (stroking) in 129, 130
  friction in 129, 130
  general 145-156
    of back 152-156
    of chest 150, 151
    of lower extremity 147-150
    of upper extremity 145-147
  general considerations 137
  indications for 135, 136
  introduction 129
  kneading (petrissage) in 129, 130
  mechanical vibration in 134
  metabolic effects of 134
  movements in 129-135
  neuromuscular effects of 133, 134
  percussion (tapotment) in 129,
    130
  petrissage (kneading) in 129, 130
  physiological effects of 131-135
  rationale of 129-138
  stroking (effleurage) in 129, 130
  tapotment (percussion) in 129,
    130
  technique of 139-156
  vibration in 129-131
Mechanical vibration in massage 134,
    135
Medicated baths 110-113
Medicated steam bath 96-98
Metrorrhagia, cold sitz bath for 42
Mild fever therapy, Russian bath for
    94
Mills, C. A. 1
Minerals, absorption of, by body 124,
    125
Mineral water, increased specific
    gravity, buoyancy, and hydro-
    static pressure of 124
  nebulized, in treatment of respira-
    tory diseases 125
Mitchell, G. K. 132, 133
Moist heat, effects of penetration of 6
Moor, F. B., and Carter, R. 8